Praise for the first edition

The gallstone-friendly diet is through the typical outpatient experience of problems with gallstones. Whilst ultimately surgery to remove the gallbladder is the only effective treatment for gallstones, the treatment pathway does involve avoiding those foods that trigger the symptoms in the early stages and whilst awaiting an operation. The recipes presented in this book provide useful guidance on how to follow a very low-fat diet – the traditional dietary modification suggested for gallstones.

I was particularly amused by the description of the patient-surgeon interaction and I think this reflects the fact that this is the commonest GI operation performed in the UK and therefore something we surgeons take for granted, not always appreciating that it is the first time for our patients. However, it is important that you and your surgeon together decide whether an operation is right or not for you as, even when the symptoms seem to fit many of the criteria for gallstones, they are such a common finding on scans, we always have to bear in mind that there might be something else going on. Having that understanding with your surgeon is an important part of any shared decision to undergo an operation. However, if the dietary steps mentioned in this book help you ahead of surgery, it is highly likely you will have a good outcome from the operation itself. To the same end, the gallstone-friendly diet may help you in your own personal gallstone journey. Good luck.

James Hopkins FRCS, Upper GI & Bariatric Surgeon
Lead for Emergency GI Surgery, North Bristol Centre for Weight
Loss, Metabolic & Bariatric Surgery, Bristol, UK

Juliet Sullivan recounts her personal story in a very honest way. She takes you through her surgery and out the other side. Unfortunately for her, she spent five months suffering from her gallstones before having her gallbladder removed. Fortunately for us, as a result of this wait she has produced a wonderful selection of recipes that are less likely to initiate pain than are standard meals. This is a truly helpful read, but if you've got gallstones, get an operation soon!

Giles J Toogood, Professor of Hepatobiliary Surgery
University of Leeds, Leeds, UK

I had little understanding of the struggles that are associated with the gallbladder before reading this book. Juliet Sullivan does a brilliant job of enlightening her audience with the facts that are necessary for understanding gallstones. Additionally, the recipes contained in this book serve as a really useful guide for anyone struggling with the dietary issues associated with gallstones. Considering that gallstones are a serious illness, Juliet Sullivan uses her humour to address the elements of unease and fear that can be associated with a diagnosis, and to assist those who struggle in navigating the lifestyle changes that will be needed. All in all, I give this book a 5/5. Fantastic job!

Nicole Irvine, Canada

I love Juliet's humour and wit. As I am dealing with gallbladder issues, this book is perfect timing as I have had no idea what to expect. I have information now to help me understand what I am dealing with. Thank you

Lorelei, Texas, USA

Juliet Sullivan's *The Gallstone-friendly Diet* is a humorous tale about her experience with gallbladder disease. You'll find yourself sympathising, laughing and gaining knowledge. Her personal anecdotes leave you with a sense of causal connection, and an understanding of how one manages with such a disease. The recipes are simple, with easy to follow instructions and tasty! If you are feeling nervous about this condition, look no further than this book to help you through it. This wonderful book leaves readers assuaged, yet hungry for more!

Mariam Nagem,
Surrey, Canada

Juliet's style is both humorous and informative. She makes you feel as though you are getting advice from a close friend. Unlike typical medical self-help books, this one will have you laughing, engaged... and making delicious gallbladder-friendly food!

Donna Moore
Canada

An excellent and amusing book with all the facts you need.

Veronica McQuade
Haywards Heath, UK

the gallstone-friendly diet

Everything you never
wanted to know about gallstones
(and how to keep on their good side)

Second Edition

JULIET SULLIVAN

With a Foreword by Iain Cameron, MD FRCS

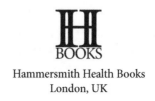

Hammersmith Health Books
London, UK

This second edition first published in 2019 by Hammersmith Health Books – an imprint of Hammersmith Books Limited
4/4A Bloomsbury Square, London WC1A 2RP, UK
www.hammersmithbooks.co.uk

The information contained in this book is for educational purposes only. It is the result of the study and the experience of the author. Whilst the information and advice offered are believed to be true and accurate at the time of going to press, neither the author nor the publisher can accept any legal responsibility or liability for any errors or omissions that may have been made or for any adverse effects which may occur as a result of following the recommendations given herein. Always consult a qualified medical practitioner if you have any concerns regarding your health.

British Library Cataloguing in Publication Data: A CIP record of this book is available from the British Library.

Print ISBN 978-1-78161-162-3
Ebook ISBN 978-1-78161-163-0

Commissioning editor: Georgina Bentliff
Designed and typeset by: Julie Bennett of Bespoke Publishing Ltd
Cover design by: Madeline Meckiffe
Cover photograph: © Stockcreations, Shutterstock
Index: Hammersmith Books Ltd.
Production: Helen Whitehorn, Pathmedia Ltd
Printed and bound by: TJ International Ltd, Cornwall

A note from the author

This book is intended to provide a light-hearted account of my own personal experience with gallstones. However, I do realise that this is a serious subject and I do not mean to trivialise the condition. I have tried to find humour in a situation that was not really at all humorous. I hope it makes you laugh, even if you are suffering from this truly horrible and distinctly unfunny illness.

The book also aims to give you ideas for what to eat as well as recipes for low-fat meals that hopefully will be gentle on your gallstones. But, despite my bold claims, I am not an expert. I am merely telling you what worked for me; hopefully it will also work for you too. I would urge you to use this book as a guide; one that might help you navigate the minefield of a gallstone-friendly diet. Good luck. You're going to need it. I shouldn't have said that, sorry.

Juliet

Acknowledgements

Thank you to my unofficial editor, Karen, for her unpaid editing and relentless support throughout my various operations and chaotic life; to my husband, 'Eel', for supporting every hare-brained idea I have ever had, including the one to write this book; to my two amazing children, 'Irrek' and 'Mail', for reasons too many to mention but mostly because they are who they are; to my friend Mia, for friendship, support and love for the past 25 years; to my 'nurses', who are so much more to me, but whose nursing/friendship skills are very welcome in my life – Mum, Tony, Catriona and Veronica. I am lucky enough to have friend/ nurses in Canada too; they will get a mention in my next book.

CONTENTS

Contents

Part II
Gallstone-friendly recipes

Contents

Contents

APPENDICES

Foreword

As a doctor who deals with hundreds of patients per year with gallstones, I find this book gives a fascinating perspective on the effect of gallstones on the life of every patient I meet with this problem. I have had four operations myself in the last 15 months and my appreciation of this book has been enhanced by my own experiences with the NHS and the mental challenges facing patients on the day of surgery and during their recovery. Just because people you know have had a similar operation and tell you how quickly they recovered, does not guarantee that your operation and postoperative recovery will follow a similar pattern. Thousands of patients every week in the NHS, undergo 'routine day case surgery', but it is vital that all healthcare workers realise that, for every patient, an operation is a major life event. I am from a non-medical background and remember vividly my father having a double hernia operation when I was 12 years old; he spent the next 25 years telling anyone who would listen, in detail, about his experience.

Gallstones are present in around 20% of the adult population, being commoner with increasing age. Most people with gallstones are unaware that they have them, until the first attack of pain that is. The description in this book of the first attack of severe gallstone pain certainly is accurate; most of my patients, including women who have had a normal vaginal delivery of a baby, will describe it as the worst pain they have ever experienced. After a severe attack of such pain, the recommendation is that patients are put on a waiting list for surgery to remove their gallbladder and given advice regarding a low-fat diet. You can imagine my surprise when, after five or six similar such conversations on a Friday morning ward round with patients admitted the previous day with gallstone pain, I return to the ward at lunchtime to find some of them eating deep-fried fish and chips. There is much we can do in the coordination of healthcare and better dietitian input is essential for this group of patients, especially as many will have to wait for several months before their gallbladder is removed.

There is some evidence for removing the inflamed gallbladder in the acute phase of the illness, although the realities and pressures of the modern NHS ensure that most people admitted with severe gallbladder pain are treated with antibiotics and analgesia initially. After discharge, a low-fat diet is recommended (with relatively little information given) and patients are either seen in a surgical clinic to consent to surgery or placed directly onto a pooled waiting list. Many people will wait up to six months for their procedure, under the constant threat of the pain flaring up again at any time; this frequently occurs in patients on the waiting list, with up to 30% requiring a second hospital admission before their operation.

This book is really helpful for patients with gallstones on many levels. It gives a realistic account of the severity of the pain, the thoughts going through patients' heads on the day of surgery, the likelihood of only meeting your surgeon and anaesthetist on the day of the operation, and the minefield that is 'a low-fat diet', which undoubtedly reduces but does not eliminate completely the risk of a further severe flare of symptoms. I think this book gives a fascinating insight into living with gallstones prior to definitive treatment, especially as this is the commonest problem patients have in my clinical practice. The author's saying that she knows what she should eat, but is not particularly good at following this through, is something that many of us can identify with in various aspects of our life.

Mr Iain C Cameron, MD FRCS
Clinical Lead, Hepatobiliary Surgery
Nottingham University Hospitals, UK

PART I

My gallstone journey
and everything I
learned on the way

My gallstone journey

Referring to my experience with gallstones as a 'journey' may be slightly misleading. It might suggest that I spent the six months waiting for my cholecystectomy enjoying a carefree, exotic existence, during which I encountered nothing less than a frivolous whirlwind of joyful fun and frolics. It may surprise you to learn that those six months were, in fact, less full of joy and more full of shit.

It was the kind of journey you might liken to driving 5000 miles alone on a twisting, pothole-littered, empty road, encountering blood-thirsty bandits around every corner.

I hope I have conveyed to you how I feel about my gallstone journey.

I won't bore you with the details. Actually, I lie. That's exactly what I'll do! We all love chatting about our own ailments, don't we? This is my story, so if I want to bore you with the details I will. But I'll be brief, because I feel like you're already quite bored.

I had always been an advocate of healthy eating. That doesn't necessarily mean I always ate healthily; it just means I advocated it. I love food. I have always loved food. And I'm English, so, let's face it, my diet had consisted of many things that didn't necessarily fit with my healthy-eating obsession. When I say obsession, I mean that in a very loose and general sense. It was more like a hobby; a part-time hobby; one that I would indulge every few weeks, perhaps. I'm rambling, like an out-of-control walking enthusiast who has lost their way on the moors.

To clarify: I was very good at knowing what I should be eating, and occasionally I did eat it. But mostly I ate things I knew I shouldn't. So that's got that little confession out of the way. It won't surprise you to know that I had spent most of my adult life being ever so slightly chubby.

I'd actually put on around five kilos every 10 years since I'd hit my twenties. Before all this gallstone crap happened to me, I was on track to weigh around 250 kilos by the time I was 100. That may not be strictly accurate; I'm not great at maths. Plus it's completely irrelevant as I probably won't make it to that ripe old age anyway.

Anyway, on a warm August afternoon nearly two years ago, I was busy indulging my part-time healthy-eating hobby. I was at a beach picnic with my sister and her family, and I was munching my way through a chicken salad. The salad had an oily dressing, but it was *olive oil*. So, healthy! I may or may not have had some chocolate afterwards.

Around 20 minutes later, suddenly and without warning, a sharp pain ripped through my chest, rendering me speechless. I was gasping for breath. It didn't last long, but it was scary, and it left a kind of lingering cramp in my chest that remained for the rest of the day. I put it down to indigestion, mainly because I wanted to swim in the sea and having a serious medical condition probably would have meant I couldn't do that.

That night, I was awoken from a deep slumber by another stabbing chest pain, and this time I was terrified. I was sure it was a heart attack; it was that painful. And in the middle of the night, with nothing to distract me, it seemed a bit more serious than it had before. It lasted for eight hours.

That was my first visit to A&E.

After hours of scans, blood tests, probing, prodding and back-passage-administered pain relief, I was sent home with a note for my GP that read: 'This woman is a pathetic wimp and/or a delusional hypochondriac.' Or at least that's what I deduced, as at a hastily arranged appointment with said GP, she concluded there was nothing wrong with me and sent me scurrying away without any suggestions as to what might have caused the eight-hour explosion of agony in my abdomen. Like it was normal. Or that I had imagined it.

Two weeks later, I went out for a lovely little lunch with my other sister. Once again, I chose a healthy option: tuna salad! How much healthier can you get? (Quite a lot, it turns out, if you have gallstones.) The salad was laden with good, healthy fats: olive oil dressing, almonds, walnuts and avocado. In retrospect, I was asking for it. I just didn't know what I was asking for.

Full disclosure: I also had a Diet Cola. Look, I know this is bad; it's actually akin to downing a litre and a half of cyanide, or so I read somewhere, but I was trying my best not to drink wine at 2:00 pm on a Friday afternoon. In my warped, uninformed little mind, Diet Cola was a healthy alternative.

Note: Diet Cola will not cause a gallstone attack because it has no fat content, but apparently all carbonated drinks are bad for gallbladder disease – notwithstanding the terrible things Diet Cola consists of.

Another note: I have not been able to face a Diet Cola drink since that fateful day, as the sight of that bubbling black temptress instantly conjures up images of the nightmare that was to transpire during the events that ensued.

The events ensued as follows: an hour after lunch, I was screaming in agony and bent double with chronic stomach pains. Shortly after that, I found myself writhing around on the floor with what can only be described as the stomach-ache from hell. It was like nothing I had ever experienced before. And I had once given birth to a giant-headed, ten-pound baby with *no pain relief*.

I phoned The Husband. These were my exact (okay, slightly edited) and very loud words: 'Get home now, and bring some Gaviscon with you!' Hilariously, I thought I had indigestion. I am not sure if it is possible for indigestion to be that bad, but (for the sake of anyone who ever plans to eat anything ever again) I really hope not.

The Pain eventually subsided. When I say subsided, I mean it skulked off into a dark corner, where it sat rubbing its hands together, cackling a comically evil laugh, and plotting its next onslaught.

I didn't have to wait long for The Pain to come creeping out of its hiding place. The Pain, you will notice, has by now taken on a life of its own, with its own name (I apologise for not being able to come up with something a little more original), and its own, sadistic, cruel personality.

This time, I was at an AA meeting.

'Ah!' you're thinking, 'this explains it! She's only got herself to blame. Obviously, years of alcohol abuse have led her to this illness. Now she's a reformed alcoholic and she is paying the price!'

But no, you're wrong!

It's my mother who is a reformed alcoholic, so there! I am not even close to being reformed.

Mum had asked if I would attend a meeting with her to learn about the AA programme and to show support. I reluctantly (because I felt not-quite-right, like I knew The Pain was preparing an imminent attack) went with her. The meeting was held in a large church hall and was packed. It was Friday night, prime time for AA meetings. The only seats we could find were at the front.

I really did not feel well, but I thought to myself, 'It's only an hour. I can do it.'

At 7:00 pm, the meeting started. Two people who were sitting at a table in front of us started speaking earnestly and passionately. One of them was crying. She was telling a story about how alcohol had almost killed her, and how AA had saved her. This stuff is gritty and real and is not to be taken lightly. The rest of the room was captivated and there was an awed silence. Except, of course, for the noises coming from my stomach – a kind of bubbling, gurgling, rumbling sound. And from my mouth – a muffled, embarrassed, moaning sound.

My mum shot me a sideways look of anger, which was quickly replaced by concern when she saw how pale I was. 'Are you okay?' she whispered... and a chorus of angry AA-ers hissed, 'Shhhhh!'

The Pain started poking around inside my tummy; then it travelled into my shoulder, my side, my back – anywhere it could find a space to inhabit. I bent double on my chair.

'Let's go,' Mum said. A loud tut came from behind us.

'No,' I said.

Leaving would have meant walking past a room of one hundred angry pairs of eyes; I didn't want to move.

The person speaking in front of us stopped speaking, and with the tears still fresh on her cheeks, she simply stared at me. At that moment, The Pain made a push for glory.

It was too much for me to bear. I cried out, got up, and hastily ran to the back of the hall, with Mum following behind.

A roomful of people were left to conclude that I was having some kind of reaction to my first day of abstinence. Or I was just plain drunk.

'I am not an alcoholic!' I wanted to shout, but this would not have endeared these people to me, I realised.

Outside, in the grounds of the church, I collapsed onto the grass in absolute agony. To the Friday night after-work crowd who were streaming past, this did not look good.

The Husband was summoned again, and he came racing to my rescue like an untrained paramedic, all helpful questions like: 'What have you eaten?' and 'Do you think you have appendicitis?'

I did think I had appendicitis, actually. It's one of those diseases that we all know about; not like *gallstones*; who's ever heard of that?

Again I found myself in A&E. This time, the triage nurse whisked me through the coveted double doors (where the doctors live) as soon as I got there. I have discovered that triage nurses don't like it when patients are screaming in the waiting room.

After again being prodded, poked, scanned, X-rayed and relieved of most of my blood supply, I sat in a room with best-friend, Mia, beside me, waiting to receive the diagnosis. A doctor arrived, her face barely visible above the giant file she carried: the hastily compiled results of my tests. The doctor introduced herself, glanced at my file and then pronounced three little words I had not been expecting: 'You're not pregnant.'

'Well, that's a huge relief,' I said, though I had no idea I'd even taken a pregnancy test. I realised that, due to the dramatic screaming and crying that had accompanied my arrival, they had concluded, quite naturally, that I was in labour.

The doctor went on to explain that lurking somewhere inside me was not a baby, but a collection of nasty little stones that were causing me the worst pain imaginable. 'How could a few tiny stones cause so much pain?' I wondered. (If you are wondering this too, all will be revealed later in the book.)

It would seem that when I took over my dad's business, Brighton Stone, my body had taken it literally. 'I know,' said my gallbladder, the day I inherited it. 'So she never forgets how lucky she is to own 17 tonnes of rocks, let's give her a few piles of rocks *inside* her body as well.'[1]

1 This sentence will not make any sense to you, but it will be explained later. Bear with me.

It was all a bit of a shock, especially when the doctor calmly announced: 'You'll go on a waiting list to have your gallbladder removed, but until then you cannot eat anything that contains fat.'

I must have turned a deathly shade that matched the ashen hospital walls, as my brain skipped right past the bit about life without a gallbladder, and instead started furiously contemplating life without chocolate, roast dinners and chicken korma! What would weekends be without the comfort of a Friday night spag bol, or a Sunday morning full English?

I turned to Mia with tears in my eyes. I was in shock.

Mia calmly turned to the doctor and asked, 'Can she still drink wine?'[2]

---

2 The doctor smiled knowingly and said, 'Yes.' Silver linings and all that.

Why I am now an expert who has written a book

I am not a doctor; nor am I a dietitian or a chef. So what gives me the right to write a recipe book – or indeed any kind of book – advising you on what to eat if you have gallstones?

Simple. I am now a self-proclaimed expert on all things gallstone-related. I accept that when asked, 'What do you want to do when you grow up?' as a youngster, I might not have replied, 'I want to traverse the mysteries of the gallbladder; discovering the truth about gallstones and conquering the world they inhabit,' but then I got gallstones.

I also admit that just a mere two years ago I didn't know what a gallbladder or gallstone was. It turns out I'm a fast learner.

My desire to learn quickly came from a desire never again to experience the truly horrific pain of a gallstone attack. I feel like that pain has taught me so much. In a way, I should be thankful for it.

I searched, in vain, to find a cookbook that would give me a selection of zero-fat or low-fat, gallstone-friendly recipes to follow. There were none. So I set about creating my own. I slaved over a hot laptop as well as stove; I researched, concocted and experimented for almost six months so that you don't have to.

Although I already understood healthy eating, I soon discovered that eating little or no fat is a whole different ballgame.

In my BG (before gallstones) days, I don't think I ever gave a second – or even a first – thought to the amount of fat in anything. I would happily consume fish and chips washed down with a glass of full-fat milk,[3] followed by apple pie and clotted cream, all within the space of an hour.[4]

Following the diagnosis, my diet was totally dictated by what would or wouldn't cause an attack.

As someone who has never successfully followed a diet, I was forced to undergo 'the gallbladder diet', which produced results Weight Watchers could only dream of. The weight just dropped off me. I lost nine kilos in five months. I know what you're thinking... Weight Watchers will probably be wanting my number.

Okay, if I'm honest the weight didn't so much drop off me as drip slowly away; painfully, agonisingly, ridiculously slowly.

During the time I was waiting for my operation, I didn't eat a single biscuit, cake, chocolate bar, egg or morsel of red meat. Not a single ounce of oil of any kind passed my lips. I consumed no nuts, butter or cream.

What I did do was make sure I was never hungry. I don't deal well with hunger. It makes me feel angry and depressed and resentful; like I'm not really living my life as it should be lived. Which is mostly eating. So I spent a lot of time developing clever ways to eat that didn't send me into toe-curling, foetal-position-inducing spasms.

---

3 That's a lie. I haven't consumed a glass of milk with a meal since I was seven years old.
4 I'm no doctor, as I've already mentioned, but I'm beginning to wonder if this kind of eating behaviour might possibly explain my subsequent medical condition.

I did lose weight, but I probably would have lost more had I not been so obsessed with food.

And I definitely would have lost more had Mia not asked that fateful question: 'Can she still drink wine?' In my deepest, darkest days, when I felt disgruntled with the world because I was a stone-infested loser whose diet and life were in turmoil, I found salvation in the fact that I could still indulge in some light alcoholic beverage consumption (which is, I believe, quite fattening).

In the interests of complete honesty, my name is Juliet, and I am …very partial to a glass of wine.

A diet and life in turmoil

When I say that my diet and life were in turmoil, I am not exaggerating for dramatic effect. For starters (no longer an option for me!), I am an eater-outer. Eating in restaurants is one of my favourite things to do. Have I already mentioned how much I love food?

I sat through two adult-children's birthdays, three house parties, a Christmas Eve, Christmas Day, Boxing Day and New Year's Eve – not to mention 22 weekends – without being able to eat 'properly'. When I went to restaurants during this time, I had to embarrass my family and friends by taking the waiter or waitress aside to explain why I couldn't eat their establishment's perfectly good food. I then had to ask them to beg the chefs to make me something delicious using ingredients they didn't have.

This would invariably end up with me drinking too much wine while jealously watching everyone else as they consumed beautiful dishes of flavourful deliciousness, which I coveted and they carelessly took for granted. Occasionally, the kitchen would produce a perfectly edible meal (actually this only happened once, in Canada), but mostly the food was – to put it mildly – bland. I have thus deduced, rather cleverly I feel, that kitchens must use a lot of oil and butter in their cooking.

At one pub, renowned for its burgers, the waitress looked at me as though I had lost my mind when I asked, 'Is there anything on the menu that's cooked without fat, oil or butter, but still tastes delicious?' On that occasion, my dinner was a pile of carrot and celery sticks.

One kitchen refused point blank to make me anything at all on the grounds that they wouldn't accept responsibility for my inevitable death after consuming their food. It's highly unlikely that I will ever return to this restaurant.

So, you see, my diet is a sad reflection of my life in general: unusual and evoking pity wherever I go.

My unusual, pity-evoking life

To really get you feeling sorry for me, I have to take you back to 2003.

Back then, I was living a perfectly nice life in my hometown of Brighton. I had a husband and two kids, aged four and 13. I owned a lovely little house in a trendy, up-and-coming area, and I worked a cushy part-time job as a legal secretary.

But no, that wasn't good enough for me! It turns out I'm a needy, ungrateful princess who wants more. I must have more! (Which is probably why I have ended up with less... a lot less.) But I digress.

One evening, after too many G&Ts and a meeting with my accountant, I decided to sell everything and emigrate to Canada. That is the very simplified version. (You can read the full story in my next book.)

The bits I have left out are quite important though: mainly that my husband Eel[5] had grown up in Canada, and had a whole life and family there that he had left behind to live with me.

So in March 2003 we found ourselves moving our family 5000 miles away to a suburb of Vancouver, where we built a new life. We bought a big, beautiful, brand new house, and we had a really nice suburban family thing going. I trained to become a real estate agent, The Husband started a successful stone-laying business, and the kids grew up healthily and happily.

But there was one problem: me. I was perpetually homesick. I spent a ridiculous amount of time and money flying back and

5 I have cleverly disguised my family members' names as they have expressed a desire not to be publicly gossiped about within these pages.

forth between the two countries. I had never really been able to let go of my connection to Brighton and to my family there. This way of life caused two more problems: debt and indecision.

Fast-forward 12 years to 2015, and my family had found itself at a crossroads. Daughter, Irrek,[6] then 25, who had always struggled with the pull of England, moved back to the UK. She found a good job and started building a new life for herself in Brighton. Our son, Mail,[7] graduated from school in Canada and decided to go to university in England. My dad was seriously ill in England. Our debts were piling up. All this conspired to push us into a momentous decision: to move back to the UK. It felt like the time was right.

We sold our big, beautiful house in Canada and packed our lives away. The same day our house sale was completed in Canada, we had a flight booked to take The Husband, The Son, The Dog, The Cat, our six suitcases and me back to England. To nothing. We no longer owned a home. We no longer had a base. Our family instantly became untethered and fragmented. As I write this, I realise how crazy it all was. It was mad behaviour. For me, it was based primarily on an emotional pull to avoid any regret around not being there for my dad when he was dying. But the move was financial suicide.

We rented a place to live in Brighton and started to build yet another chapter of our lives. I took over my dad's stone-selling business, Brighton Stone (as mentioned earlier), mainly because he wanted me to, but it was a mistake. I sell houses – and books, hopefully – not stones.

And then, one by one, my family members left me to return to Canada, starting with The Husband. We had kind of known that

6 & 7 Once again, I have cleverly disguised my family members' names as they have expressed a desire not to be publicly gossiped about within these pages.

would happen, as his business, life and family were there; we just hadn't really thought it through. We're still together, but spend most of our time apart.

The Son, now aged 18, decided he didn't want to study in England after all. He returned to Canada after four months.

And then The Daughter met a boy. Said boy was travelling to Australia and she persuaded him to stop off in Canada. She subsequently flew there to meet him and never came back.

I was left alone in England, committed to a business I knew nothing about. I was around when my dad died, and that was hugely important, but the major consequence of that series of decisions was an empty bank account. The truth is that it cost us several hundred thousand dollars.

But it's not the money I mourn. It's my family life. My husband and kids live on the other side of the world, while I live alone with my dog (the cat pissed off as soon as we got here; hopefully she's not also trying to get back to Canada). I spend my time running a failing stone business, walking an ageing, resentful dog, and having operations. (This is the second I have had since returning to England. More of that in my third book. I am sure you cannot wait.)

The four of us fly way more than we should, especially me. I spend my life in a state of perpetual jetlag, for which I am working on a cure. Look, I need money, okay?

So I think we're all caught up. Now you know how sad my life is and why you should: a) feel desperately sorry for me, and b) send me a few quid.

The day of surgery

I actually had two days of surgery, because I am greedy like that – one is never enough for me! – though the first time around I managed to hang on to my gallbladder. It was a cold Monday morning in December and I had been instructed to arrive at the hospital at 7:00 am sharp. I have never been anywhere at 7:00 am sharp, and obviously the thought of it sent my body into sheer panic. I had returned from a Canada trip two weeks earlier especially for this surgery but, along with terrible jetlag, I picked up a nasty cold that stayed with me until the day I arrived at the hospital.

The Husband was flying in specially for the big day. We sound so bloody exotic, don't we? His flight landed at 11:00 am, perfect timing to avoid the real drama of the day (me being somewhere by 7:00 am) and just in time to arrive at the hospital to find a gallbladder-free wife. The plan was for him to look after me post-surgery and run the business while I was in recovery. We sell Christmas trees and obviously, being early December, this was a fairly busy time for us.

My sister, Karen (I'm bored with cleverly disguising names), kindly volunteered to drive me to the hospital after I had calmly asked her: 'How the hell am I going to get to the bloody hospital by 7:00 am?' When she arrived to collect me from home, I was a snivelling, snotty mess. The cold I had been battling for two weeks was at its full-blown worst.

The admissions nurse took one look at me and demanded that I leave the hospital immediately and return only when I was no longer a threat to civilisation. Well, that's what her eyes conveyed, anyway. What she actually said was: 'You are not fit to have an operation.' I wittily replied, 'I didn't know I had to be

fit to have an operation. Seems like something of an oxymoron.'
And we laughed.

We didn't laugh. *I* laughed.

Two things really upset me about this whole experience:
1) I had got somewhere at 7:00 am for no reason
2) I was clearly going to miss out on an opportunity for The Husband to tend to my every need for the following two weeks.

The other (actual) day of surgery

They gave me another surgery date in January. This time, The Husband had to stay in Canada for 'work reasons'. I left him at the airport in Vancouver after a lovely (fat-free) family Christmas, and we both cried. I knew I was coming back to face a tough, painful, lonely month, and he knew he was a lucky bastard for not having to deal with it. I think his were tears of joy.

This time they gave me an afternoon slot. It was all so much nicer. When I say 'nicer', I mean it was nicer than, say, sitting in your accountant's office waiting for an audit from the taxman. I spent a leisurely morning contemplating the day ahead. I couldn't eat or drink, so I sat on my bed for three hours doing nothing, staring at nothing in particular, and wondering what I had done in my life to deserve this. Everything just seemed so wrong. I texted The Husband to say that this was the lowest point of my life. I felt it was important that he share my misery from 5000 miles away.

I should mention here that I know how lucky I am. I have very supportive family and great friends around me in England. I have a life in two countries; two families and two sets of friends. But it's the division of my life that is so hard. The constant, gnawing feeling that something, or someone, is missing. In tough times, it just becomes a little harder to bear. And I have a tendency towards drama, hence the dramatic text to The Husband.

His reply? 'Everything is temporary.' Simple and blunt – some would say cold and heartless – but true.

I sat in the hospital waiting room alone, sadly clutching a plastic bag that contained my dressing gown and slippers. I was shaking uncontrollably. (Is there any other kind of shaking?) I contemplated feigning a cold, fainting, or just running for the exit. But I was brave, even though I would shortly be lying like a slab of meat on an operating table, my fate in the hands of someone whose nickname was probably the Butcher of Surrey, or the Gallbladder Snatcher.

A nurse walked me down to the operating theatre. We chatted as we walked, and to take my mind off the fact that I was about to be opened up and relieved of one of my organs, she asked me various questions. My favourite was: 'What's the first thing you're going to eat after your surgery?'

I really liked this approach, which made me look at the positives of this mostly negative situation.

'Probably everything!' I replied truthfully. I had been having fantasies about cream cakes and chicken stew for weeks.

'I told my husband the next time I saw him I'd be as fat as a house!' I said. It was a throwaway comment; it wasn't meant to illicit questions and subsequent tales of woe and abandonment.

'What do you mean, *when you see him next*?' she asked. 'Where is he?'

I should have just said, 'Afghanistan'. It would have been so much easier to explain. But instead, my surgery had to be delayed by three hours while I shared my convoluted marital situation with the nurse.

As she was leaving my bedside, the nurse referred to my state of affairs as 'heart-wrenching', and as soon as she left I started to cry. I suddenly felt very sad and alone.

This nurse had told me that, as well as being a nurse, she was a long-haul flight attendant *and* had three small children. I told her I admired her, and I do. I'm in awe of her. I would have liked to be her friend, despite her intrusive line of questioning, but there's no way she has time for me in her life.

Shortly after this, my surgeon approached the bed and introduced himself. He was nice enough, but too casual, I thought, for someone who was soon to be intimately manhandling my insides. I wanted to know more about him, but I wasn't given the chance to find out. He seemed reluctant to chit-chat and, unlike the nurse, didn't even try to be my friend.

After that, I was wheeled into a room where I met my anaesthetist and her sidekick. I especially liked my anaesthetist, an older lady who saw how nervous I was and inspired confidence by saying things like: 'In 30 years I have never killed anyone off!'

She also paid me a compliment as she was inserting something sharp into my vein. I'll take a compliment wherever I can get one, but it was hard to appreciate this one as my teeth were chattering wildly and I was having terrible thoughts, mainly about death. I really do not enjoy surgery.

'I noticed you're 51. You really don't look it,' she said.

I sort of smiled and tried to convey my appreciation of positive age-related comments as I put my life in this woman's hands.

She and the sidekick seemed to be having an argument about something as I drifted off to sleep. I wanted to stay awake to listen, but maybe it was best that I didn't. I'll never know now what they were quibbling about. Maybe he thought I looked older than 51. Rude!

And so eventually it was all over, and you will be relieved to learn that I survived. It was a miracle! My new friend the nurse had said something about gallbladder surgery being equivalent to a 'beautician giving a pedicure', which was weird and confusing, but I still wanted to be her friend.

I suppose her point was that it's routine, and that recovery is not a big deal.

I think the nurse and I might have been heading for our first falling-out. Because it *was* a big deal. For me, anyway.

I personally know four people who have had the operation, and all four claim they were out of bed by day two after the op. One, a good friend, even said that she was back at work within a day of leaving the hospital, but I have since realised she is a pathological liar.

Post-surgery

Here are a few observations and tips for how you might be feeling in the days that follow your surgery:

1) As soon as you wake up, your first thought will be, 'I can eat food again!' You will be desperate to savour the delights of anything containing fat, while marvelling at how pain-free you are. (However, in reality, you won't want to eat much. In fact, you won't be hungry for a few days. I nibbled on a biscuit as soon as it was offered to me because I felt obliged to do so after six months of biscuit-free living, and I was curious to see if I could even stomach such a fat-laden thing without any ill-effects. It didn't taste good. But I hadn't actually left the recovery room yet; it was probably too soon. And of course, you're not really pain free. You are coming round from a general anaesthetic and are pumped full of beautiful painkillers. As soon as these wear off, you will know pain again; it's just that it will no longer be caused by your gallbladder... unless of course the surgeon has forgotten to actually remove it.)

2) As soon as you get home, you will be tempted to jump on the scales. You are feeling certain at this point that doing so will make you feel smug, gorgeous and very, very thin. I made the mistake of doing this, expecting to have lost at least three kilos. After all, I hadn't eaten for a whole day while I was otherwise busy having an operation, and on top of that I'd had a very heavy organ removed. (I knew it was heavy because it was full of stones!) Sadly, the scales reported that I had gained two kilos. I later learned (through some hasty Googling) that during the op they pump you full of gas, which stays in your body for a week and causes bloating, farting and extreme pain in your shoulder. So don't get on the scales for at least a week. And don't look in the mirror! You will resemble a pasty, swollen, giant pufferfish.

Other tips for post-surgery

1) Don't plan to go back to work any time soon. I had actually made plans to go to work four days after my op. In retrospect, I feel silly about this. I was still struggling to get out of bed at that point.

2) Expect some bruising. No one warned me about this, and I was shocked to see that my stomach looked as though it had done 10 rounds with Mohammed Ali.

3) Don't assume (assuming you have had keyhole surgery) that your recovery will be any different from open surgery. I have no idea what the recovery from open surgery would be, as I had keyhole, but I do know I expected it to be a walk in the park. Keyhole surgery sounds so simple! A few tiny incisions here, a little squirt of gas there, a little tugging, and voila – one less organ to worry about! It wasn't a walk in the park, and in fact I couldn't walk in the park for two weeks.

4) Don't encourage your 20-year-old son, who is 5000 miles away in Canada, to text you to say that he is seriously ill. As you lie in bed contemplating your life's choices, your dire situation and the fact that you cannot get out of bed let alone get on a plane to go and comfort your sick son, your recovery will be probably delayed by several days. In retrospect, *this* was my lowest point. But it will probably be different for you. I hope so.

A rolling (gall)stone gathers no moss

I recovered fully from the op after around six weeks – a little longer than I had expected, but to be honest, in the end I was just grateful that it was all over.

It took a little while longer for the mental anguish to disappear. (You may remember, I am a little dramatic.) But I do still feel a little strange; like I have something missing. I keep marvelling at how our bodies function, and that even when a surgeon removes part of them, they still continue to work.

In all honesty, I had briefly contemplated not having the surgery at all, for several reasons:
1) I'm a bit of a baby.
2) I read lots of advice online that recommended not having the surgery and suggesting that the gallstones can be treated naturally.
3) Treating the gallstones naturally involves trying to flush them out of your body. I found a cure that involved drinking a cocktail of lemon juice and olive oil (more on that later, you will be delighted to know). Olive oil was my biggest trigger and enemy, so I decided not to put myself through a self-induced attack.
4) See point 1.

I'm glad that I finally went through with it because the surgeon told me (after the op) that a large stone was blocking my bile duct. And I have no idea what that means, but it sounds bad and it makes me think that I made the right decision.

Living in fear of a gallstones attack is no fun. The worst example of this level of no-fun is when I flew business class between London and Vancouver (on a very cheap standby flight, I might

27

add, in case you think I'm lying when I say I need money). To be seated on a plane for almost 10 hours while you are offered amazing, free food, and not to be able to accept it, is nothing less than torture.

Knowing that I will never again experience the hellish pain of an attack is worth the significantly less-hellish experience of an operation.

Although I will probably never again eat red meat, cheese or high-fat meals, I pretty much can eat a 'normal' diet again, which is great but also terrifying. I don't want to put those hard-lost nine kilos back on. My plan is to eat a similar diet to the one I have trained myself to live on over the past six months, with two differences:

1) I will add some healthy fats: olive oil, nuts, seeds, avocado etc.

2) When I eat out, I will eat more – a lot more – than raw vegetables.

So, happily, I can report that my diet is no longer in turmoil.

As for my life, well that's another story.

I'm not joking. That is actually another story. Available soon on Amazon.

Almost everything you never wanted to know about your gallbladder and gallstones

If you sit around all day wondering what causes gallstones, what they are made of and what your gallbladder is actually for, I would love to explain. As I mentioned earlier, I didn't know six months ago what the gallbladder was, where it was in the body, or what it was for. But now I know the following, which I can share with you.

What is the gallbladder?

The gallbladder is a pear-shaped organ that sits just below the liver. It is linked to the liver by the hepatic biliary ducts and then links through to the first part of the small intestine (the duodenum) via the bile duct and the 'common' bile duct. A diagram makes it much easier to understand that – see Figure 1 on the next page.

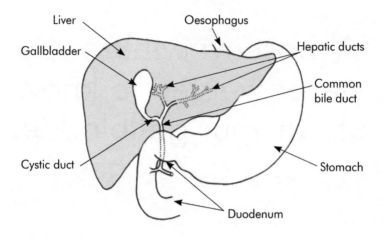

Figure 1: The gallbladder in relation to the liver and gut

What are gallstones?

Gallstones occur when bile creates stones that most commonly contain lumps of fatty (cholesterol-like) material that has solidified and hardened. The stones can be as small as a grain of sand or as big as a golf ball.

There are three types of gallstones – cholesterol stones, which account for 80% of gallstones; pigment stones, which are composed of bilirubin, a brownish-yellow substance found in bile and made from broken-down haemoglobin (the red pigment in blood that carries oxygen); and the least common stones, known as 'mixed composition stones', which contain varying proportions of cholesterol, bilirubin and other substances, such as calcium carbonate, calcium phosphate and calcium palmitate.

Sometimes just a few small stones are formed; other times a great many. In my case, many stones had formed, including a giant one. I'm a bit competitive, so what I am trying to say is I had more stones than you, so there.

Do many people get gallstones?

About one in three women and one in six men form gallstones at some stage in their lives, and they become increasingly common with age. Around 12-15% of the population in both the UK and the USA have gallstones. However, not everyone who has gallstones will experience their pain. It is thought that only around 20% of people with gallstones will ever know about it. But that equates to a lot of people in a lot of pain.

Gallstones are known to be more prevalent in North America, Europe and Australia, and are less prevalent in Africa, India, China, Japan and Egypt. This suggests that a Western diet – high in refined carbs, trans fats and dairy – could well play a part in the formation of gallstones.

As well as a generally unhealthy diet, the risk of forming gallstones increases as a result of:
- Pregnancy
- Obesity
- Diabetes
- Smoking
- Rapid weight loss
- Having a close relative with gallstones
- Taking certain medicines, such as the contraceptive pill.

Look out for the Four Fs!

According to common belief within the medical field, if you fall into any of the following categories, you are at a higher risk of developing gallstones:

Female

Fat

Fertile

Forty.

In my extensive research for this book, I discovered that the famous gallstone sufferers of the world include the Dalai Lama. So, you see, even llamas can get gallstones.

Wait. I got a bit confused, sorry.

To clarify: the famous gallstone sufferers of the world, other than me, include the Dalai Lama (a man!), Andy Warhol (a man!), the singer Pink (female but not fat, not 40!), Eric Clapton (also a man!) and the Princess of Denmark (female but also not fat, also not 40!).

The fact is, there are many factors involved in developing these nasty little stones, not least of which is something to do with genetics. Thanks, Mum.

Before those heady gallstone days, I didn't give my gallbladder a whole lot of thought. Although there was that one time years ago when I was contemplating my general health, and I decided to start looking after, cherishing and appreciating my gallbladder.

That's not true; no-one has ever done that – until they got gallstones, that is. This organ does not rank on the same 'popularity' scale as, say, the heart, or the liver, or even one of the other organs we can do without – the appendix, or the tonsils (why do we have so many pointless parts?).

But, wait – *is* the gallbladder pointless? And if not, how come surgeons are so happy to whip it out? Firstly, we have to understand what the gallbladder actually does.

What is the gallbladder for?

The gallbladder collects and stores bile, made by the liver as a result of its many detoxification processes. It then releases the bile into the small intestine when food enters from the stomach. This helps with the digestion of food because the gallbladder contains bile salts and other substances that neutralise the acid contents of the stomach as they arrive in the duodenum and emulsify and break down fat.

The bile duct, which connects the gallbladder to the small intestine, can become blocked by gallstones, making it difficult for bile to be released from the bile duct. This is what may cause symptoms - the extreme pain, bloating, nausea and vomiting associated with a gallstone attack.

Can we live without the gallbladder?

I really hope so, as I no longer have one. To be serious for a minute, the answer is, 'Yes'! But.

According to Dr Sandra Cabot MD, in her book (co-authored with naturopath Margaret Jasinska ND) *Save Your Gallbladder Naturally and What to do if you've already lost it*:

> *A significant number of patients who have had their gallbladder removed continue to suffer with pain and digestive problems. According to a study published in the British Journal of General Practice it was found that having the gallbladder surgically removed does not always relieve upper abdomen pain.* *

> *Without a gallbladder, your liver continues to manufacture*

*Berger MY, et al. Is biliary pain exclusively related to gallbladder stones? A controlled prospective study. *British Journal of General Practice* 2004; 54: 574-579

bile, but there is no longer a place to store it or concentrate it. Therefore bile continually slowly trickles into the intestines. If you eat a fatty meal, you will not be able to secrete a large enough amount of bile into your intestines, therefore the fat will be poorly digested. This means many people experience diarrhoea, bloating, nausea or indigestion.

Not digesting fat well means you will not be able to digest essential fatty acids, including omega 3 and omega 6 fats, which are necessary for good health. It also means you'll have a hard time absorbing fat-soluble vitamins, such as vitamins D, E, A and K. A lot of the antioxidants in vegetables are fat soluble: lycopene, lutein and carotenoids are all fat soluble. If you don't produce adequate bile, you will not be adequately absorbing these life-saving compounds from foods.

Some common symptoms of poor fat digestion are dry, brittle hair; dry skin and premature aging of the skin; weak nails and painful joints. Essential fatty acids are important for optimal brain health, therefore low mood, anxiety, depression and impaired cognitive function are all possible manifestations of poor fat digestion.

Once your gallbladder has been removed:

• *Keep your intake of dairy products and grains to a minimum, or avoid them altogether. Dairy products (milk, cheese, ice-cream, yoghurt) worsen all cases of gallbladder disease and liver disease and they are very difficult to digest. Food intolerance is a common cause of gallbladder problems, and there is research that links gluten intolerance with gallstones. A good reason to keep your intake of grains low is to reduce the risk of developing a fatty liver.*

• *Take a good quality liver tonic, such as Livatone. The herbs*

St Mary's thistle, dandelion root and globe artichoke leaves all increase bile production and bile flow. Taurine is an amino acid necessary for bile production. This should help to make you feel more comfortable after a meal, and should reduce the risk of stones forming inside your liver.

- *Take an ox bile supplement. A lack of bile can produce symptoms such as bloating and indigestion after meals, light coloured stools, diarrhoea, fatigue after meals and nutrient deficiencies. Taking a good quality ox bile supplement with each meal is wonderful for completely eliminating these symptoms in most individuals.*

- *Take a digestive-enzymes supplement. The majority of people who develop a gallbladder problem have suffered with poor digestion for many years. If your stomach and intestines are not in optimal health, they will not send signals to your gallbladder, telling it to contract properly. Irritable bowel syndrome, dysbiosis, small intestinal bacterial overgrowth and candida overgrowth are common in people with a gallbladder problem. If you have had your gallbladder removed, you may continue to suffer symptoms due to those conditions. These digestive problems also cause insufficient digestive enzyme production. Taking digestive enzymes in supplement form helps to restore good digestive health and reduces symptoms of indigestion.*

- *Eat some good fats and avoid the bad fats. Your doctor may have recommended you follow a low-fat diet after having your gallbladder removed. This is not necessary and in fact it is harmful. Your body desperately needs good fats and I recommend you include moderate quantities of extra virgin olive oil, avocados, coconut milk and oil, nuts and seeds in your diet.*

- *You may need a vitamin D3 supplement. People with compromised liver or digestive function are often vitamin D deficient. Exposure of your skin to the sun's UVB rays enables your body to manufacture vitamin D. However, this process occurs in your liver and kidneys. People with a sluggish liver often do not manufacture vitamin D adequately. Therefore it's a good idea to get a blood test and take a supplement; 5000 IU of vitamin D3 is a safe and effective dose for most people, but it's best to be guided by your own doctor.*

• *Include some bitter and sour foods in your diet. They should help to improve your digestion and make it easier to tolerate good fats in your diet. Suitable bitter and sour foods include lemons, limes, radicchio lettuce, chicory, endive and dandelion leaves.*

• *Find out if you have a food allergy or sensitivity. If you still experience pain or digestive problems after having your gallbladder removed, there is a very good chance you are eating foods your body considers harmful. The biggest culprits are gluten, eggs, onions, pork, corn and soy. You may need the help of a naturopath or nutritionist to help you identify your food sensitivities.*

Prevention of gallstones

If you are reading this book, I would assume that you already suffer from the charming little nuggets of delight. But, if there are some people in your life who don't have gallstones (and I really hope there are), then you may wish to impart the following information to help them in what I must insist should be their new anti-gallstone-formation quest. They will thank you. And me.

Here are some suggested ways to ward them off:

- Number one is diet. Avoid crash diets or low-calorie diets. Eat good sources of fibre (raw fruits and vegetables, cooked dried beans, peas, wholegrain cereals and bran, for example). Avoid eating too many fatty foods but do not avoid fat altogether. Limit sugar intake, both refined and natural. Lower your carb intake – better still, cut out refined and processed carbs (white flour, pasta, cakes and pastries) altogether.

- Studies have shown that a moderate consumption of olive oil as well as legumes, fruits and vegetables may lower your chances of developing gallstones.*

- Lecithin: Many natural health practitioners believe that lecithin – a natural substance found in foods such as soy beans, kidney beans, cooked Brussels sprouts and broccoli – may help reduce cholesterol, which in turn may prevent gallstones. Lecithin is also said to help reduce blockages. Soya lecithin powder may reduce cholesterol absorption and lower LDL ('bad') cholesterol when added to fat-free foods. Even though most people get plenty of lecithin in their normal diet,

* Barré A, Gusto G, Cadeau C, Carbonnel F, Boutron-Ruault MC. Diet and risk of cholecystectomy. A prospective study based on the French E3N cohort. *Am J Gastroenterol* 2017; 112(9): 1448-1456. doi: 10.1038/ajg.2017.216. Epub 2017 Jul 25.

supplements are available in tablet or liquid form. (Check with your doctor or nutritionist before taking lecithin supplements.) Note: Lecithin is an emulsifier, which is one of the functions of bile, so it is also beneficial to take lecithin after a cholecystectomy – if taken with fatty foods, the body can process them better and extract essential fatty acids.

- Lose weight (if necessary): If you are overweight, you will likely have a higher level of cholesterol in your bile, which can increase the risk of developing cholesterol stones. Losing weight can reduce this risk, but remember that losing weight quickly is a contributing factor in gallstone formation. So do it gently – 1 to 2 pounds (0.5-1 kilos) a week is recommended.
- Stay active: Not only does exercise help keep your weight in check, but there is some evidence that physical activity may help prevent the formation of gallstones by improving bile flow. Aim for 30 minutes of moderate-intensity activity – where you feel warm and slightly out of breath – five times a week.
- Smoking has been shown to increase the risk of gallbladder disease, according to the British Liver Trust. So, if you smoke, try to stop.

Options for treating gallstones

I was made to feel like I didn't have a choice in treating my gallstones. (I love referring to them as 'my gallstones', like they are an old boyfriend. Though I have to say, things didn't end well for that particular boyfriend.)

I was told, 'You need to have your gallbladder removed,' and that was that. No discussion; no question and answer session; no apologies; nothing. But the reality is that surgery does not have to be the default solution.

Many doctors will employ a 'wait and watch' approach if your gallstones are not symptomatic; but if they are, the options are generally as follows:
- Symptom management through nutritional and lifestyle changes to help prevent gallstone pain
- Surgery
- Medical intervention, such as pain killers and antispasmodic medication when needed
- Attempts to dissolve the stones or reduce their size, using the chemicals ursodiol or chenodiol (although the stones can recur)
- The natural approach, which includes the 'gallbladder flush' – not for the faint-hearted (in my opinion).

In her book *Overcoming Gallstones*, Dr Sarah Brewer gives some information on this:

The gallbladder flush

The gallbladder flush is a folk remedy said to promote the passage of gallstones. The 'flush' typically involves fasting for 12 hours and then drinking a large amount of olive oil and lemon juice.

Usually, a laxative and/or enema is also used. This produces diarrhoea, abdominal pain and the passage of multiple green, brown, yellow or black spheres which resemble gallstones.

However, analysis shows that these hardened blobs are not stones, but bile-stained 'soaps' produced by an interaction between the ingested oil and other ingredients of the flush. They are often produced in quantities far greater than could be stored in a gallbladder and could be told apart from real stones because the 'soap' blobs:

- *are soft, waxy or gelatinous whilst real gallstones are either hard or dry and crumbly in texture*

- *float on toilet water as they are largely composed of oil, whereas genuine gallstones would sink*

- *do not have the sharp facets produced when real gallstones rub against each other in the gallbladder*

- *can be cut cleanly with a knife (unlike real gallstones) and often have bright green translucency that is never seen with real stones*

- *disintegrate over time unless frozen, whereas gallstones are stable.*

There is no scientific evidence that the gallbladder flush works, and it may in fact be harmful. Even if the large amount of oil did promote ejection of a small gallstone into the cystic duct and out into the bile duct, this would be immensely painful and debilitating and would probably involve admission to hospital for investigations and pain relief.

Other natural options which I did not try but are said to help gallstone symptoms and may warrant further investigation include black seed oil and turmeric. I would recommend testing these in small quantities though before committing to regular consumption.

Foods that are said to aid the secretion of digestive enzymes and promote bile secretion include:

Raw beetroot juice
Radishes
Limes
Apples
Pears
Grapefruit
Chamomile tea.

Again, though, it might be a good idea to test these foods in small quantities, and try them out individually rather than consuming them all in one go.

Why do I need a gallstone-friendly diet?

Whether you have opted for natural treatment, or you are waiting for surgery, you will need to watch your diet. Although experts believe that a no-fat diet can be harmful, it does seem to be universally accepted that cutting down on fat intake does reduce the likelihood of a gallstone attack, as, without fat, the gallbladder will not be stimulated to release bile into the small intestine.

Here are some easy ways to cut down on fat:

- Avoid processed foods and cook from scratch wherever possible. This will give you control over how much fat goes into your food.
- Check labels for high-fat content.
- Bulk out meals with vegetables and pulses. For example, you could make a gallstone-friendly Bolognese by replacing the meat with lentils, kidney beans and mushrooms.
- Use oil spray when cooking – this will become your new best friend.
- If you are cooking anything that is sticking to the pan, use a few drops of water rather than oil. This is known as 'steam frying'. I have also used wine to 'fry' food. Wine adds moisture as well as flavour. Most of the alcohol will burn off in the cooking process.
- Make your own dressings using low-fat yoghurt, lemon/lime juice and herbs. (More on this later in the book.)
- Remove all visible fat and skin from meat and choose leaner cuts. I avoided all red meat while I waited for my op, but I did eat some chicken, turkey and fish.
- Avoid eating out, but if you do, ask the kitchen to dry-roast, grill or bake your food. Some will agree to do this. Avoid sauces, dressings and gravies. Expect to resent everyone in the restaurant who is eating 'normally'.

Some personal recommendations

Suggested supplements

Apple cider vinegar

A quick Google search (not recommended – but this is unlikely to stop you!) will reveal a whole load of advice on how to alleviate gallstone pain, and high on the list is usually apple cider vinegar. There is no supported evidence to suggest that it alleviates pain or (as is sometimes claimed) dissolves the stones, but apple cider vinegar does have anti-inflammatory properties, which in turn can help most digestive-related diseases.

Instructions for use: Mix two tablespoons of good quality apple cider vinegar with a small glass of organic apple juice.

I drank this every day because it felt like the right thing to do. I cannot say for certain whether or not it helped, but it certainly didn't hurt.

Omega-3 capsules

In the absence of much fat in my diet, good or bad, I opted for an omega-3 capsule every day. I also took an evening primrose oil capsule daily, as it contains omega-6. It is important to balance omega-3 with omega-6, ideally on a 1:1 ratio. A balanced combination of the two essential fatty acids promotes good health and keeps inflammation in the body in check.

Psyllium husks

Psyllium husks are also a great help with gallstones. Psyllium cleanses the colon, which is important, since constipation is linked with gallstone formation. You should take 1-3 teaspoons in 300 ml of water each morning, and again last thing at night.

Magnesium

I am middle-aged (even though I don't look it, according to my lovely anaesthetist), so magnesium is important, not just for bone health and calcium absorption, but magnesium also helps in the metabolism of food and synthesis of fatty acids and proteins.

Probiotics

A good daily probiotic is essential for a healthy gut. My gut is not healthy, but one day it will be again. Although I found no recommendations advising the consumption of probiotics to help with this condition, I felt that I needed to address a generally unhealthy gut. Probiotics are said to boost the immune system, help ward off infection and reduce the population of harmful bacteria in the gut – which all seemed like a good idea. I took a probiotic containing *Lactobacillus rhamnosus GG* (LGG) which is said to help the digestive system work better generally.

Vitamin C

Studies* have shown that taking regular supplements of vitamin C may be associated with a reduced prevalence of gallstones.

Milk thistle

Milk thistle (also known as *Silymarin marianum* and St Mary's thistle – see page 151) is a prickly composite herb from the Mediterranean region and has been used extensively in traditional folk medicine to treat liver and gallbladder diseases. Milk thistle is sometimes used to shrink gallstones, but it is essential that you speak to your doctor before embarking on a milk thistle regime.

Peppermint tea

Peppermint contains menthol, a soothing compound that promotes pain relief. It can be used to ease stomach pain, improve digestion and relieve nausea.

*Gustafsson U, Wang FH, Axelson M, Kallner A, Sahlin S, Einarsson K. The effect of vitamin C in high doses on plasma and biliary lipid composition in patients with cholesterol gallstones: prolongation of the nucleation time. *European Journal of Clinical Investigation* 1997; 27(5): 387-391. PubMed PMID: 9179545.

A note about exercise

I am a 'serial occasional' exerciser. I have been through times in my life where exercise was an everyday part of my routine, and times when the treadmill was gathering dust in the corner.

Prior to my gallstones nightmare, I had been indulging in some light yoga as well as a bit of circuit training, but I quickly gave it up based on the logic of 'any old excuse'. I think the key here is: if you feel okay, do it.

I rarely felt fit enough to exercise during the five-and-a-half months of my gallstone days. I felt like a pain in my chest was always lurking, and I just never felt like myself. Other than walking every day, I avoided anything strenuous. I have read that yoga is a good option and, based solely on that, I would highly recommend it.

Also, I would always, in any situation, for any reason, recommend swimming. Swimming is the best low-impact, stress-relieving, health-promoting exercise out there. I just didn't feel like doing it.

Everyone is different, though, and hopefully you're not as lazy as me.

Food!

And now, for the exciting part: food! In the following pages I will list the recipes that I found, adapted, or just plain made up to suit this new regime. These recipes all rely on eating a minimal amount of fat.

If you do not have gallstones (or after you have got rid of the nasty little darlings), these recipes can still be used but should not be wholly relied upon as part of a balanced diet. Good fat should be part of your diet if you are gallstone- or gallbladder-free.

Top tip: Eat little and often!

PART II

Gallstone-friendly recipes

The fat index

If I was a bit cleverer, I would list the fat content of each recipe in this book. But I am not that clever, and I am a bit lazy. Also, I want you to think about the foods you are eating, because all of our journeys are different. So, it's all about you, and to help you I have simplified things. (You're welcome!)

Each recipe has been allocated a star rating (listed below), not according to how delicious it is – because all my recipes are delicious! – but according to the approximate fat content. I have found 5 grams per serving (max) to be the magic number.

But I have also found that I can personally eat small amounts of fish, chicken and turkey, and this will push the total fat content up. Your tolerance may be different. The point of these recipes is to show you how to cook using the minimal amount of fat.

⭐⭐⭐ ULTRA-LOW FAT (approximately less than 3 grams of fat per serving)

⭐⭐ LOW FAT (approximately less than 5 grams of fat per serving)

⭐ LOWISH FAT (approximately 5 grams of fat per serving plus the protein)

BREAKFAST

Good old fashioned porridge ✪✪✪

I have rediscovered porridge and you will too! It is not only low fat, low calorie and delicious, but it is really good for you.

I am sure you don't need a recipe for porridge, but here are some tips to make it gallstone-friendly:

- Use skimmed milk or water instead of full fat milk, although it is worth noting that skimmed milk is higher in sugar content than some milk alternatives – see table below
- Add a combination of berries, bananas and fat-free or low-fat yoghurt – so healthy.

Top tip: I add soya-based chocolate dessert or chocolate soya milk to mine for a touch of indulgence – though it does make it more like a dessert than a breakfast.

Fat/sugar content of milk and milk alternatives

Per 100ml	Approx fat content	(of which saturated)	Approx sugar content
Cow's milk (full fat)	3.6 g	2.3 g	4.6 g
Cow's milk (skimmed)	0.1 g	0.1 g	4.8 g
Goat's milk	3.5 g	2.4 g	4.3 g
Unsweetened soya milk	1.8 g	0.3 g	4.3 g
Unsweetened almond milk	1.1 g	0.1 g	0.0 g
Coconut milk	0.9 g	0.8 g	2.0 g
Hemp milk	2.8 g	0.3 g	1.8 g
Oat milk	1.5 g	0.2 g	4.0 g
Rice milk	1.0 g	0.1 g	4.0 g

Low-fat pancakes ✪✪✪

In this recipe I use a sugar alternative, just to keep calories down and because it's best to avoid sugar generally. You can of course use real sugar if you like, or omit it altogether if you don't want your pancakes sweet.

Ingredients

- 75 grams (½ cup) gluten-free flour
- 1 tbsp stevia (or ½ tbsp sugar)
- ¼ tsp baking powder
- ¼ tsp salt
- 1 large egg white
- 118 ml (½ cup) skimmed milk
- ¼ tsp vanilla extract
- coconut or olive oil cooking spray, or water for steam frying

Method

Mix the flour, baking powder and salt in a large bowl. Add the stevia or sugar.

Whisk the egg white, milk and vanilla extract in a small bowl.

Add the wet ingredients to the dry and stir well.

Heat a non-stick frying pan for a couple of minutes on high, then squirt a few sprays of the magic oil spray into the pan, (or a few drops of water if you are steam frying).

Immediately pour your batter into the pan and cook until bubbles form and the edges appear dry, then flip and cook for another 1-2 minutes.

To serve:

Add blueberries, bananas, raspberries and pomegranate seeds. Drizzle with honey for a little extra indulgence.

Veggie omelette ✪✪

Tricky one this, as technically the omelette is made from eggs
and eggs are one of the enemies. I found that if I used egg whites
only (which are pure protein), everything was good.

Ingredients

- egg whites from 2 eggs
- bunch of spring onions, chopped
- 1 red pepper, chopped
- 1 green pepper, chopped
- 2 tbsp skimmed milk
- salt and pepper
- coconut or olive oil cooking spray, or water for steam frying
- parsley

Method

Mix the egg whites with the chopped onions and peppers.
Add the milk and seasoning.
Heat a non-stick frying pan for a couple of minutes on high, then
squirt a few sprays of the magic oil spray (or water) into the
pan.
Immediately add the omelette mixture and cook until firm
underneath.
Place under a hot grill to cook the top for 2-3 minutes, until it's
nicely browned.
Sprinkle with parsley and serve.

Top tip: If you're feeling indulgent, you can top the omelette
with smoked salmon if you like it and find no problems with
eating it – I found I could tolerate it but it might be too oily for
some.

The good old English fry-up (sort of) ⭐

I found myself facing Christmas whilst dealing with this gallstone situation, and so some compromises had to be hastily made to accommodate my family's Christmas Day tradition of full English breakfast followed by full turkey roast (more of that later). This is my version of the 'gallstone fry-up'. This recipe serves one, because you will likely be the only one eating like this.

Ingredients

- 4 small potatoes, peeled and halved
- coconut or olive oil cooking spray
- 2 good-quality low-fat veggie sausages – my favourite are Cauldron Vegan Mediterranean sausages (3.9 grams of fat for 2)
- 4 cherry tomatoes
- 4 mushrooms
- egg white from 1 egg
- 2 tbsp skimmed milk
- 200 g (7 oz) tin of baked beans

Method

Parboil the potatoes.
Heat a roasting pan in the oven for 10 minutes.
Add 4-5 pumps of the oil spray to the roasting tin.
Drain the potatoes and add to the roasting pan; roast for 25 minutes.
Put the sausages in a roasting pan in the oven and cook for 15 minutes.
Heat a frying pan, then add a few pumps of the spray and lightly fry the tomatoes and mushrooms.
Meanwhile, mix the egg whites with the milk, add salt and pepper, and scramble in a non-stick saucepan.
Heat the beans, and then serve all together.

Home-made muesli ✪✪✪

I have always made my own muesli, but in the old 'Before Gallstones' (BG) days I would include nuts and seeds. This is the low-fat version.

Ingredients

- 128 grams (1 cup) dry porridge oats
- 2 tbsp water
- 2 tbsp orange juice
- 2 tbsp lemon juice
- 1 apple, sliced
- handful of blueberries and raspberries
- handful of pomegranate seeds
- 1 banana
- 1 tbsp raisins
- drizzle of honey, optional

Method

Mix the oats with water and leave overnight. This draws out the starch from the oats.

Before serving, mix in the orange juice, stir, and then add the fruit and the lemon juice.

Drizzle with honey if you want extra sweetness to counteract the lemon juice.

Apple sauce oatmeal muffins

Because this recipe uses olive oil, it is recommended that you eat one muffin at a sitting, as the fat content is around 3.5 grams per muffin.

Ingredients

- 112 grams (1¼ cups) dry porridge oats
- 160 grams (1¼ cups) whole wheat flour
- 1 tsp baking powder
- ½ tsp bicarbonate of soda (baking soda)
- ¼ tsp salt
- ½ tsp cinnamon
- 255 grams (1 cup) unsweetened applesauce* see recipe on page 56
- 120 grams (½ cup) low-fat buttermilk (obtainable from most supermarkets)
- 100 grams (½ cup) brown sugar
- 1 tbsp olive oil
- 2 tbsp egg white, lightly beaten
- 75 grams (½ cup) raisins

Method

Preheat the oven to 200°C/400°F.
Line a 12-cup muffin tin with paper cases or spray with coconut or olive oil cooking spray.
In a large bowl, combine the oats, flour, baking powder, bicarbonate of soda, salt and cinnamon.
In a medium bowl, combine the applesauce, buttermilk, sugar, oil and egg white.
Make a well in the centre of the dry ingredients and add applesauce mixture.
Stir until just moist.
Fold in the raisins.
Fill the muffin cups two-thirds full.
Bake for 16-18 minutes or until springy to the touch.

Unsweetened apple sauce ✪

Ingredients

- 4 medium cooking apples
- 235 ml (1 cup) water
- ½ tsp cinnamon
- 1 tbsp lemon juice

Method

Peel, core and chop the apples (or you can leave skins on if preferred).
Add the apples to a saucepan with the cinnamon and lemon juice.
Add half of the water, and then top up with more during cooking as needed (to get the desired consistency).
Bring to the boil, reduce the heat, cover and then simmer gently for 25-30 minutes until apples are soft.
Mash it all together using a potato masher or hand blender.
Leave to cool and transfer to a jar.
Store in the fridge until needed. It should keep for up to 7-10 days.

Berry smoothie ✪✪✪

This is substantial enough to be a complete breakfast.

Ingredients

- 200 ml (1 cup) skimmed milk
- selection of fresh or frozen berries: blueberries, blackberries, raspberries
- 1 banana

Method

Blend until smooth.

Kale and cucumber smoothie ✪✪✪

Ingredients

- handful kale
- 200 ml (1 cup) skimmed milk
- 1 banana, peeled and chopped
- ¼ cucumber, chopped
- handful of frozen berries

Method

Tear the kale leaves from their stalks and place into your blender.
Add all the remaining ingredients to the blender and blend until smooth.
You can substitute a large handful of spinach for the kale or, for a super-food smoothie, add it to the kale to make a kale, cucumber and spinach smoothie. You may need to add some extra liquid.

Mango and honey smoothie ✪✪✪

Ingredients

- 200 ml (1 cup) skimmed milk
- ½ mango, peeled and pitted
- 1 banana, peeled and chopped
- handful of frozen berries
- ½ tsp honey

Method

Throw it all in the blender and blend until smooth.

Other low-fat breakfast ideas

Note: Watch your sugar intake! A high-sugar diet leads to insulin resistance which leads to high cholesterol which leads to gallstones, so the following are not necessarily long-term gallstone-friendly suggestions.

Toast and jam ✪✪✪

Don't mock. I am just giving you options. I was elated when I realised I could eat toast and jam. Just make sure you pick a low-fat bread (most bread has around 1 gram of fat per slice, but some has more). Obviously, don't add butter or margarine. I spent a lot of time searching for good-quality, natural-sugar jams and marmalades (they have no fat but sugar content can be high).

Note: Choose gluten-free bread if you have a sensitivity to gluten, or low-carb bread to bring the carb content down.

Crumpets ✪✪✪

Crumpets are a good, filling alternative to bread; you can put a tiny scraping of low-fat butter on if you want to; or if you prefer not to risk it, stick to jam or marmalade, or a very low-fat cream cheese.

Plus

Beans on wholemeal toast
Scrambled egg on wholemeal toast (made with egg whites
    and skimmed milk)
Fat-free yoghurt with berries and/or honey
Fresh fruit salad

Breakfast

Smoked salmon with wholemeal bread
Vegetarian sausages with baked beans (check for fat
   content)
Weetabix with skimmed milk and banana
Bran flakes with skimmed milk and blueberries
Cornflakes with skimmed milk and banana
Banana bread: see recipe on page 116.

LUNCH

Veggie skewers ✪✪✪

Ingredients/equipment

- 6 cherry tomatoes
- 1 courgette (zucchini), sliced
- 1 onion, quartered
- 1 yellow pepper, sliced
- 1 red pepper, sliced
- 4 mini corn-on-the-cobs
- coconut or olive oil cooking spray
- 2 skewers

Method

Load skewers up with the veg.
Give everything a light spray with the cooking spray.
Place under a pre-heated grill and grill for 10 minutes or until
    everything is crisp and perfect.

Top tip: Add prawns or chicken for a great dinner option –
obviously be aware that this will increase the fat/cholesterol
content.

Curried sweet potato ✪✪✪

Ingredients

- 1 small sweet potato
- 1 tsp curry powder
- salt and pepper

Method

Bake the potato for 1 hour or until soft inside.
Scoop out the potato, mix with the curry powder and add salt and pepper to taste.
Return to the potato skin and serve.

Tomato salad ✪✪✪

Ingredients

- 114 grams (4 oz) mixed ripe tomatoes
- salt and pepper
- pinch of oregano
- 4-6 tbsp red wine or balsamic vinegar
- 1 clove garlic
- 1 red chilli, seeded and chopped

Method

Slice some of the tomatoes in half, leave others whole – it mixes things up a bit.

Place them all in a colander with a good pinch of salt.

Give them a toss, season again and give a couple more tosses for good luck.

Leave the tomatoes in the colander on top of a bowl to stand for around 15 minutes, then discard any juice that has come out of them.

Transfer the tomatoes to a large bowl and sprinkle over the oregano.

Make a dressing using the red wine or balsamic vinegar (or a mixture of both), the garlic and the chilli.

Drizzle the tomatoes with enough dressing to coat everything nicely.

Top tips:

- Use lots of different types of tomatoes, to give this salad the WOW factor.
- Also… adding salt to the tomatoes will really bring out their flavour, so don't skimp on this step.

Sandwiches

I don't think you need to avoid bread completely, but you do need to limit it, and always buy whole grains. Stay away from white bread.

As for sandwich fillings, obviously stay away from butter and spreads... but you do have some options as listed below:

Cucumber and tomato
Mushroom and spinach
Prawn and salad
Tuna (in water) and salad
Smoked salmon and cucumber
Cucumber
Tuna, celery and apple
Turkey and salad
Chicken (no skin) and salad
Banana.

Top tip: I also discovered chutneys and sauces – most of which have no fat content. They add an interesting touch of flavour to your sandwich – but watch the sugar content.

Veggie curry topping ✪✪✪

Ingredients

- coconut or olive oil cooking spray, or a few tablespoons of wine, or water for steam frying
- 1 onion, chopped
- 2 cloves garlic, crushed
- 2½ tbsp curry powder
- 2 tbsp tomato purée
- 1 x 400 gram (14 oz) tin chopped tomatoes
- 1 vegetable stock cube
- 350 grams (2 cups) frozen mixed vegetables
- 340 ml (12 fl oz) water
- salt and pepper to taste
- chopped fresh coriander (cilantro) or parsley to garnish

Method

Heat a saucepan over a medium heat for 2 minutes, then give a few pumps of the cooking oil spray (and/or the wine/water).

Sauté the onion and garlic until golden.

Stir in the curry powder and tomato purée.

Cook for 2 to 3 minutes.

Stir in the tomatoes, vegetable stock cube, mixed vegetables, water, salt and pepper to taste.

Cook for approximately 20 to 30 minutes until the veg are well done (not crunchy).

Sprinkle with fresh coriander (cilantro) or parsley prior to serving.

SOUPS

Carrot and coriander (cilantro) ✪✪✪

Ingredients

- coconut or olive oil cooking spray, or a few tablespoons of wine or water for steam frying
- 4 large carrots, peeled and roughly chopped
- 1 onion, roughly chopped
- 900 ml (1 ½ pints) vegetable stock
- large bunch fresh coriander (cilantro), roughly chopped

Method

Heat a saucepan over a medium heat for 2 minutes, then give a few pumps of the cooking spray, (or wine / water).

Sauté the onion and carrots for a few minutes until the onion has softened.

Pour in the vegetable stock and add the coriander (cilantro).

Bring to the boil and cook until the carrots are tender – around 10 minutes.

Remove from the heat and allow to cool slightly.

Purée the soup until smooth, using a hand blender or food processor.

Serve with a small wholemeal roll.

Fat-free minestrone ✪✪✪

Ingredients

- 1 onion
- 2 cloves garlic
- 1 x 400 gram (14 oz) can plum tomatoes
- 1 courgette (zucchini)
- 1 carrot
- 1 red pepper
- 115 grams (¼ lb) red split lentils
- 1 tbsp tomato purée
- 1 tsp dried basil
- 1 tsp dried oregano
- 850 ml (1½ pints) vegetable stock
- 55 grams (2 oz) spaghetti
- salt and pepper to season

Method

Chop the onion, crush the garlic and cook together gently in enough water to cover the bottom of your pan.

Purée (or chop to a pulp) the tinned tomatoes and add to the onion and garlic.

Thinly slice the courgette, carrot and red pepper and add to the pan.

Add the lentils, tomato purée and dried herbs and mix well.

Turn the heat up until bubbling and add the stock.

Simmer for 30 minutes.

Break the spaghetti into tiny pieces and add to the soup.

Cook for a further 15 minutes.

Season and serve.

Potato and celery soup ✪✪✪

Ingredients

- coconut or olive oil cooking spray, or a few tablespoons of wine or water for steam frying
- 1 large potato, peeled and diced
- 1 onion, diced
- 850 ml (1½ pints) chicken stock
- 1 bunch celery
- ½ tsp celery salt (or sea salt)

Method

Heat your frying pan over medium heat for 2 minutes, then pump a few sprays of the cooking oil spray (or wine / water) into the pan.

Sauté the potato and onion for 3 minutes or until the onion has turned translucent.

Pour in the chicken stock and bring to the boil.

Once boiling, add the celery.

Bring back to the boil and lower the heat, then add the celery salt/ sea salt.

Let simmer for 30 minutes.

Purée the soup with a hand blender or food processor until smooth.

Curried carrot soup ✪✪✪

Ingredients

- coconut or olive oil cooking spray, or a few tablespoons of wine or water, for steam frying
- 1 onion, chopped
- 1 tbsp curry powder
- 1 kg (2¼ lb) carrots, chopped
- 1 litre (1¾ pints) vegetable stock
- 500 ml (17 fl oz) water, or as needed

Method

Heat a pan on a medium heat, and then add the cooking oil spray, (or wine / water).

Sauté the onion until tender and translucent.

Stir in the curry powder.

Add the chopped carrots and stir until they are well coated.

Pour in the vegetable stock, and simmer until the carrots are soft – about 20 minutes.

Transfer the soup to a blender, and purée until smooth (or use a hand-held blender).

Pour back into the pot, and thin with water to your preferred consistency.

Butternut squash soup ✪✪✪

Ingredients

- 1 whole butternut squash, peeled and chopped
- 1 large onion, chopped
- dash of balsamic vinegar
- dried herbs – a bit of what you fancy, such as basil, garlic, oregano, rosemary
- coconut or olive oil cooking spray, or a few tablespoons of wine or water for steam roasting
- 1.6 litres (6.5 cups) chicken stock
- salt and pepper

Method

Pre-heat the oven to 200°C/400°F.

Line a roasting pan with tin foil and place it in the oven to pre-heat.

Toss the chopped butternut squash, chopped onion, balsamic vinegar and your dried herbs together in a bowl.

Take the roasting dish from the oven and pump a few sprays of the cooking oil spray, (or wine / water) , enough to coat the bottom.

Transfer your mixture to the roasting dish.

Bake for around 25 minutes, giving it a stir halfway through.

Cook until all the veg are soft and starting to caramelise.

Place the roasted veg into a food processor with about a quarter of the stock, adding more if needed.

When smooth, pour the mixture into a large saucepan and add the remaining stock.

Simmer for around 10 minutes and add more herbs, and salt and pepper, as necessary.

Black bean and salsa soup ✪✪✪

Ingredients

- 2 x 400 gram (14 oz) tins black beans, drained and rinsed
- 350 ml (12 fl oz) vegetable stock
- 225 grams (8 oz) tomato salsa dip
- 1 tsp ground cumin
- 4 tbsp fat-free plain yoghurt
- 3 spring onions, thinly sliced

Method

In an electric food processor or blender, combine beans, stock, salsa and cumin; blend until fairly smooth.

Heat the bean mixture in a saucepan over a medium heat until thoroughly hot.

Ladle the soup into individual bowls and top each bowl with 1 tablespoon of the yoghurt and a sprinkling of spring onion.

Top tips:

- High in fibre and packed with nutrients, black beans are a healthy addition to any dish (but make sure they are thoroughly cooked as they are poisonous if not).
- If you can't find tinned black beans, use dried (but make sure to soak overnight and cook for a minimum of two hours before using).

Other low-fat lunch ideas

Beans or spaghetti hoops on toast

Toasted tomato sandwich

Vegetarian sausages with salad or baked beans (but check fat content as not all vegetarian sausages are created equal)

Vegetarian sushi (or with salmon if you can tolerate it)

Dry-roasted sweet potato fries with fat-free yoghurt dip

Tuna (in water) salad with home-made dressing (page 108 for dressings)

Spinach and black bean salad

Smoked salmon salad with home-made dressing (see page 108 for dressings)

Baked salmon fillet with salad

Smoked salmon sandwich

Smoked salmon omelette

Ham omelette (use lean ham sparingly and egg whites only)

Baked potato with baked beans

Baked sweet potato with baked beans

Baked potato with tuna (in water) and sweetcorn

Baked potato with tuna (in water) and chopped celery

Baked potato with veggie chilli (recipe page 82)

Baked potato with veggie curry topping (recipe page 67)

DINNER

Grilled fish and greens with capers and lemon salsa ⭐

Ingredients

- 4 white fish (e.g. cod, sea bass, hake, haddock) fillets, sustainably sourced
- 350 grams (2 cups) tenderstem broccoli
- 150 grams (1 cup) trimmed green beans
- 1 bunch spring onions
- coconut or olive oil cooking spray
- salt and pepper
- 1 lemon
- small bunch fresh parsley
- 1 tbsp capers

To serve:
- Lime wedges
- Steamed rice

Method

Heat the grill to high, then coat the fish, broccoli, beans and spring onions with a few oil sprays, and season well with salt and pepper.

Put the vegetables in a large shallow baking tray, reserving the fish, and grill on high for 4 minutes.

Meanwhile, for the salsa, trim the skin off half the lemon, slice the peeled lemon into thin rounds, and then cut the rounds into small wedges, discarding any seeds; put these in a bowl.

Finely chop the parsley and mix with the lemon and a few sprays of the oil.

Drain the capers, add to the lemon and parsley mixture with some salt and pepper, and mix well.

Add the fish on top of the veg, then grill for 4-5 minutes more (or longer, depending on the thickness of the fish fillets) until the fish is just cooked and the vegetables are soft and sweet.

Squeeze over the remaining lemon and serve with the salsa and lime wedges.

Veggie curry ✪✪✪

Ingredients

For the spice mixture:

- 2 tbsp cumin seeds
- 1 tbsp coriander (cilantro) seeds
- 1 tbsp cardamom seeds
- 1 tsp mustard seeds
- 4 cloves

- 2 onions, sliced
- 2 garlic cloves, crushed
- 550 ml (2⅓ cups) vegetable stock
- 1 fresh red chilli, deseeded and finely chopped
- 1 x 2½ cm (1 inch) piece fresh root ginger, peeled and chopped
- 1 tsp turmeric
- 110 gram (3.8 oz) button mushrooms
- 1 aubergine, cubed
- 110 gram (3.8 oz) cauliflower florets
- 110 gram (3.8 oz) broccoli florets
- 150 gram (5.2 oz) fat-free natural yoghurt
- salt and freshly ground black pepper
- 2 tbsp chopped coriander (cilantro) leaves

Method

Make the spice mixture by grinding all the spices together in an electric grinder or with a pestle and mortar.

Put the onions, garlic and half the stock in a saucepan; cover and bring to the boil for 5 to 10 minutes. Uncover and simmer for 20-30 minutes until the onions are tender.

Add the chilli, ginger, turmeric and ground spice mixture; cook gently for 2-3 minutes to allow the spices to release their aroma.

Add the mushrooms, aubergine and cauliflower with the remaining stock, then cover the pan and simmer for about 20 minutes.

Meanwhile, cook the broccoli separately in boiling, salted water until just tender and still green; drain, and add to the curry.

Stir in the yoghurt very gently and heat through gently on a low heat – do not allow to boil or the yogurt will curdle.

Check the seasoning and serve the curry immediately, sprinkled with the coriander (cilantro).

Chicken curry ⭐

Ingredients/equipment

- 2 onions, sliced
- 2 cloves garlic
- 4 cm /1.5 inches) ginger
- 2 bird's-eye chillis
- 4 tbsp fat-free yoghurt
- 500 grams (1.1 lb) chicken breasts or thighs, skin removed
- coconut or olive oil spray, or wine or water for steam frying
- 1 tsp ground cumin
- 2 tbsp ground coriander (cilantro)
- ½ tsp turmeric
- ½ tsp garam masala
- 2 tsp salt
- 2 x 400 gram (14 oz) cans chopped tomatoes

Food processor or blender

Method

Peel the onions, garlic and ginger and take the top off the chilli; include the chilli seeds (if you dare).

Throw it all in the blender and whizz it all up until it's finely chopped.

Put half of the mixture in a bowl and stir in the yoghurt.

Cube the chicken and add to the yoghurt mix; allow to marinate for around an hour.

Heat a saucepan or frying pan for a few minutes, then spray a few pumps of the oil spray, (or wine / water), into the pan.

Fry the half of the onion mixture not used for the marinade for 2-3 minutes, then add the cumin, turmeric, garam masala and 1tbsp of coriander / cilantro and salt.

In the blender, whizz the tomatoes, then add those to the pan and cook on a low heat for around 30 minutes.

Add the chicken and yoghurt mixture to the pan, stir and cover.

Cook for about 40 minutes.

Serve with rice or a rice alternative.

Throw a dollop of fat-free yoghurt on top to make you think you are indulging.

Sprinkle with the remaining coriander (cilantro) for maximum effect.

Prawn curry ⭐⭐

Ingredients

- coconut or olive oil cooking spray, or a few tablespoons of wine or water for steam frying
- 2 medium onions
- 2 cloves garlic, crushed
- small piece of ginger, grated (around 1 tsp)
- 4 tsp turmeric
- 2 tsp garam masala
- 2 tsp paprika
- 2-4 tsp chilli flakes of your choice
- 2 tins x 400 gram (14 oz) chopped tomatoes
- 2 tbsp brown sugar (or 1 tbsp stevia)
- 400 grams (14oz) raw prawns
- pinch of salt and pepper
- 3 tbsp fat-free Greek yoghurt plus extra dollop for serving
- 1 tbsp coriander (cilantro)

Method

Heat a saucepan or frying pan over a medium heat for 2 minutes, then add a few squirts of your best friend the oil spray, (or wine / water).

Add the onions,, garlic, ginger, turmeric, garam masala, paprika and chilli flakes and fry until the onions are soft and a nice paste has formed. Throw in your tomatoes, sugar, salt and pepper.

Cook until some of the water has reduced.

Once the sauce has thickened up a bit, add the prawns.

Cook until they curl up on themselves a bit and become completely opaque.

Stir the yogurt through; this will create a nice creamy sauce and colour.

Serve with a dollop of fat-free yoghurt and a smattering of coriander (cilantro) for that extra touch of garnish.

Veggie chilli ✪✪✪

Ingredients

- coconut or olive oil cooking spray, or a few tablespoons of wine or water for steam frying
- 1 red onion, chopped
- 1 red pepper, chopped
- 4 garlic cloves, minced
- 2 tsp sea salt
- 1 large sweet potato, cut into cubes
- 1 lime, zest and juice
- 1 400 gram (14 oz) can diced tomatoes
- 1 can sweetcorn, drained
- 2 x 400 gram (14 oz) cans kidney beans rinsed and drained
- 1 fresh jalapeno pepper, seeded and chopped
- 1 tbsp cumin
- 1 tbsp chilli powder
- 1 lime, cut into wedges (optional – for garnish)
- 1 cup chopped coriander (cilantro) (optional – for garnish)
- 500 grams (2¼ cups) brown rice (optional to serve)
- 4 tbsp fat-free plain yoghurt (optional to serve)

Method

Warm a large pan over a medium heat for 2 minutes, then coat the base thinly with the cooking oil spray, or water/wine.

Add the onion, red pepper, garlic and salt and sauté until soft – around 4 minutes.

Add the sweet potato and lime zest, and cook for another 10-15 minutes, stirring occasionally.

Add the tomatoes, sweetcorn, black beans, jalapeno, lime juice, cumin and chilli powder, and bring to a simmer, cover, and cook for 10 minutes.

Sprinkle with coriander (cilantro) (optional – for garnish)

Serve with fat-free yoghurt and brown rice.

Honey and lime chicken ✪

Ingredients

- 600 grams (1.33 lb) boneless, skinless chicken breast, cut into thick strips
- 1½ grams (¼ cup) coriander (cilantro)
- 4 tbsp lime juice
- 2 garlic cloves
- 1½ tsp honey
- ½ tsp sea salt
- ½ tsp cumin
- ½ tsp red chilli pepper flakes
- coconut or olive oil cooking spray
- 1 tbsp plain fat-free yoghurt

Method

Add the coriander (cilantro), lime juice, garlic, honey, salt, cumin, red chilli pepper flakes, and yoghurt to a food processor; pulse until a marinade/sauce is formed.

(If you do not have a food processor, just mix the ingredients together until blended well.)

Marinate the chicken in half of the mixture overnight, ideally for around 24 hours; save the remaining sauce for dipping/drizzling.

When it is ready to cook, remove the chicken and let excess marinade drip off.

Place the chicken into a grill pan.

Lightly spray with the cooking spray.

Pre-heat the grill and cook the chicken for about 4-5 minutes per side, or until cooked through.

Serve with salad or grilled asparagus and rice.

Prawn and courgette barley risotto with white wine ⭐

Ingredients

* 830 ml (3½ cups) fat-free chicken stock
* coconut or olive oil cooking spray
* 300 grams (2 cups) chopped courgettes
* 300 grams (2 cups) chopped onion
* 150 grams (1 cup) lightly pearled barley
* ¼ teaspoon salt
* 225 grams (½ pound) medium prawns, peeled and de-veined
* 235 ml (1 cup) white wine
* ¼ tsp freshly ground black pepper

Method

Bring the stock to a simmer in a medium saucepan; keep warm.
Heat a non-stick skillet over a medium-high heat and add a few
    pumps of the oil spray.
Add the courgettes (zucchini) and onion and sauté for 5 minutes or
    until tender, stirring frequently.
Add the barley and cook for 1 minute, stirring constantly.
Stir in 1 cup of the stock and cook 5 minutes or until the liquid is
    nearly absorbed, stirring frequently.
Stir in 75 ml (½ cup) of the stock plus salt and cook until the liquid
    is nearly absorbed..
Add the remaining stock, 75 ml (½ cup) at a time, stirring frequently
    until each portion of stock is absorbed before adding the next
    (about 25 minutes).
Add the prawns and cook for 4 to 5 minutes.
Stir in the white wine and pepper and serve.

Veggie spag bol ⊗⊗

Ingredients

- 1 carrot
- 1 onion
- 1 stick celery
- 1 red pepper
- coconut or olive oil cooking spray, or water / wine for steam frying
- 100 grams (2/3 cup) red lentils
- 400 grams (14 oz) tin of tomatoes
- 600 ml (1 pint) fat-free vegetable stock
- 2 tsp dried oregano
- ½ tsp ground cinnamon
- salt and pepper
- 250 grams (3½) cups spaghetti
- parsley (optional – for garnish)

Method

Roughly chop the carrot, onion, celery and red pepper.
Heat a large saucepan for 2 minutes, then coat the base with a few sprays of the oil, or water / wine.
Fry the veg for about 8 minutes until soft.
Stir in the lentils, tomatoes, stock, oregano and cinnamon.
Bring to the boil, reduce the heat, cover and simmer for 20 minutes.
Season, then simmer for a further 5 minutes.
Cook the spaghetti according to the packet instructions.
Serve with the sauce and sprinkle with the parsley.

Veggie shepherd's pie ✪✪✪

Ingredients

- coconut or olive oil cooking spray, or water / wine for steam frying
- 1 medium onion, peeled and finely chopped
- 1 large clove garlic
- 2 sticks celery, finely chopped
- 1 large carrot, thickly diced
- 300 grams (4 cups) organic mushrooms, cleaned
- 2 tsp rosemary
- 2 tsp thyme
- 150 ml water, filtered
- 400 gram (14 oz) can chopped tomatoes
- 2 fat-free vegetable stock cubes
- 100 grams (²/₃ cup) frozen peas
- 400 gram (14 oz) can green or brown lentils, rinsed and drained
- salt and pepper

For topping:
6 large potatoes (or sweet potatoes – or mixture of both), boiled and mashed with black pepper and salt

Optional: these ingredients can be added before the potatoes are added and prior to placing the pie in the oven, depending on your personal preferences and taste:

2 tbsp red wine
400 gram (14 oz) can baked beans
400 gram (14 oz) can black beans, drained
400 grams (14 oz) sweetcorn, drained

Method

Heat a large frying pan on a medium heat for 2-3 minutes and then thinly coat the bottom with the cooking spray, or water / wine.

Fry the onion and garlic until soft.

Add the celery, carrot and mushrooms, rosemary and all but a sprinkling of the thyme.

Pour in the wine (if using), 150 ml water and the tomatoes, then sprinkle in the stock cubes and simmer for 10 minutes.

Add the peas.

Tip in the can of lentils, and any other beans or ingredients (if using), then cover and simmer for another 10 minutes until the carrots still have a bit of bite and the lentils are pulpy.

Pile the lentil mixture into a pie dish, spoon the mash on top and add seasoning to taste.

(The pie can now be covered and chilled for up to 2 days, or frozen for up to a month.)

To heat:

Heat the oven to 190°C/375°F.

Cook for 20 minutes if cooking straight away, 40 minutes from chilled, or 1 hour 15 minutes from frozen, until golden and hot all the way through.

Serve with fresh green veg.

Ratatouille ✪✪✪

Ingredients

* 4 large tomatoes
* 2 aubergines (eggplant)
* 2 courgettes (zucchini)
* 2 red peppers
* 2 garlic cloves
* coconut or olive oil cooking spray, or water / wine for steam frying
* 3 tsp *herbes de Provence*
* 3 tsp dried thyme
* 3 tbsp tomato puree
* 1 tsp honey
* juice of 1 lime
* 2 tsp soy sauce
* 1 tsp chilli powder
* 2 tsp paprika

Method

Score a line on the bottom of the tomatoes, then put them in a pan of boiling water and let them sit for around 30 seconds.

Drain the water, rinse the tomatoes under cold water and then peel off the skins.

Chop them into small pieces, discarding the skins and seeds.

Chop the remaining vegetables into bite-size pieces.

Crush the garlic into a saucepan with a few sprays of your cooking spray, or water / wine, add the herbs and cook for a few minutes until bubbling, then add all the veg.

Place a lid on the pan and simmer for around 30 minutes on a medium heat, until all the veg are soft.

Stir in the tomato purée, honey, lime juice, soy sauce, chilli and paprika.

Cook it all together for a couple of minutes and then serve.

Penne perfecto ✪✪✪

Ingredients

- 125 grams (2 cups) gluten-free, wholegrain penne (or wholegrain pasta of your choice)
- 1 tsp dried oregano
- 1 tsp dried thyme
- 1 tsp chilli flakes
- 2 garlic cloves, crushed
- coconut or olive oil cooking spray, or water / wine for steam frying
- 12 cherry tomatoes
- 200 gram (7 oz) can chopped tomatoes
- 1 tbsp tomato purée
- juice of 1 lemon
- salt and pepper

Method

Cook the pasta according to the packet instructions.

Meanwhile, heat a frying pan on a medium heat for 2 minutes, then coat the base with the cooking spray (or wine / water).

Add the oregano, thyme, chilli and garlic and sizzle gently.

Cut the cherry tomatoes into quarters, then add these to the pan along with the tinned tomatoes and tomato purée; cook for around 5 minutes, until the cherry tomatoes are soft.

Add the lemon juice and salt and pepper.

Drain the cooked pasta, and then stir into the sauce.

Prawn and asparagus pasta ✪✪

Ingredients

* 1 onion
* 4 sticks celery
* 1 red pepper
* 1 bunch asparagus spears
* coconut or olive oil cooking spray and/or a glug of red or white wine, or water for steam frying
* 12-15 prawns
* 400 grams (14 oz) tomatoes
* 2 tsp dried oregano
* salt and pepper
* 250 grams (3½) cups pasta of your choice
* parsley (optional – for garnish)

Method

Roughly chop the onion, celery, red pepper and asparagus.

Heat a large saucepan for 2 minutes, then coat the base with a few sprays of the oil (and/or wine and/or water).

Fry the veg for about 8 minutes until soft.

Add the prawns and fry until fully cooked.

Stir in the tomatoes and oregano.

Bring to the boil, reduce the heat, cover and simmer for 10 minutes.

Add salt and pepper.

Cook the pasta according to the packet instructions.

Serve with the sauce and sprinkle with the parsley.

Veggie stir fry ✪✪✪

Ingredients

- 1 onion
- 4 sticks celery
- 1 red pepper
- 1 bunch asparagus spears
- a handful each of broccoli, carrots, sugar snap peas, according to your preference
- coconut or olive oil cooking spray/glug of red or white wine, or water for steam frying
- sweetcorn, peas, baked beans – whatever you fancy
- 2 tsp dried oregano
- salt and pepper
- 4 tbsp soy or teriyaki sauce (optional)
- parsley (optional – for garnish)
- wholegrain rice

Method

Chop the onion, celery, red pepper, asparagus, broccoli and carrots – and whatever vegetables you are using.

Heat a large saucepan for 2 minutes, then coat the base with a few sprays of the oil, (or wine / water)

Fry all the vegetables for about 8 minutes until soft.

Add the sweetcorn, beans or peas (if using).

Add salt and pepper.

Add the soy or teriyaki sauce (if using).

Add chicken or prawns if you fancy it (obviously will increase the fat content).

Sprinkle with the parsley.

Serve with wholegrain rice.

Sweet potato risotto ⭐

Ingredients

For the rice:

- 500 grams (2¼ cups) brown rice
- 700 ml (3 cups) water
- 118 ml (½ cup) low-fat coconut milk
- 2 tbsp apple cider vinegar
- salt

For the sauce:

- 4 large sweet potatoes
- coconut or olive oil cooking spray
- 200 ml (1 cup) water
- salt and pepper
- 1 tsp cinnamon
- 1 tbsp apple cider vinegar
- 3 tbsp nutritional yeast
- 1 tbsp ground cumin
- juice of 1 lemon
- 3 garlic cloves
- handful of fresh coriander (cilantro)
- 225 grams (1 cup) spinach

Method

Pre-heat the oven to 180°C/350°F.

Put the rice into a large saucepan with 700 ml (3 cups) of water.

Add the coconut milk, 2 tbsp of apple cider vinegar and salt.

Bring to the boil, then reduce to a simmer, cover and cook for around 40 minutes or until the liquid has been absorbed.

Meanwhile, chop 3 of the sweet potatoes into bite-size chunks, place them on a baking tray and coat them thinly in the cooking spray; then add salt, pepper and cinnamon and put the tray in the oven to cook for 30 minutes.

Peel the fourth sweet potato, cut into bite-size chunks and place in a steamer until really soft.

Once the steamed potato is cooked, add to a blender with 200 ml (1 cup) water plus the remaining apple cider vinegar, yeast, cumin, lemon juice, garlic, salt and pepper and blend until smooth.

Once the rice is cooked, stir in the blended mixture along with the roasted sweet potato chunks, coriander/cilantro, and spinach.

Allow to cook until the spinach has wilted, then serve straightaway.

Fiery fajita bowls ⭐

Ingredients

- 250 grams (1 cup) brown rice
- coconut or olive oil cooking spray or water/wine for steam frying
- 1 onion, sliced
- 1 medium courgette (zucchini), cut into sticks
- 1 red pepper, sliced
- 1 yellow pepper, sliced
- 3 medium mushrooms, sliced
- 1 tsp smoked paprika
- ½ tsp cayenne pepper
- ½ tsp ground cumin
- salt and pepper

For the simple homemade salsa:
- 2 large tomatoes, diced
- 1 spring onion, finely chopped
- 2-3 sprigs fresh coriander (cilantro), finely chopped
- salt and black pepper

To assemble:
- fresh coriander (cilantro)
- chopped spring onions
- hot sauce
- salad
- low-fat sour cream (optional)

Method

Boil the brown rice in plenty of water, until cooked to your liking (around 20 minutes), then drain.

Meanwhile, heat a large frying pan or wok over a medium heat, then thinly coat the bottom with cooking spray, and add the chopped vegetables.

Add the spices, and a pinch of salt and pepper.

Cook over a high heat, stirring regularly, for about 5-10 minutes, until the vegetables are soft.

To make the simple homemade salsa, place the diced tomatoes in a bowl with 1 chopped spring onion and a sprinkling of fresh coriander (cilantro); add a pinch of salt and pepper, and mix.

To assemble your veggie fajita bowls, serve the cooked brown rice into three bowls, top with the vegetable mixture and add the homemade salsa.

Finish with a dollop of low-fat sour cream (if using), some chopped coriander (cilantro) and spring onions, and a dash of hot sauce.

Top tip: Add prawns or chicken if you like, but remember to be aware of the added fat/cholesterol content.

Veggie winter stew ✪✪

Ingredients

- 5 carrots, peeled and sliced
- 2 x 400 gram (14 oz) cans chopped tomatoes
- 100 grams (½ cup) puy lentils
- 5 tbsp tomato purée
- 3 tsp ground cinnamon
- 3 tsp ground ginger
- 3 garlic cloves, crushed
- 5 tsp soy sauce
- salt and pepper
- 600 ml (2½ cups) water, boiled
- 3 courgettes (zucchini), sliced
- 2 x 400 gram (14 oz) cans cannellini beans, drained and rinsed
- juice of 1 lime
- 500 grams (2¼ cups) brown rice (optional to serve)

Method

Add to a large saucepan: carrots, chopped tomatoes, lentils, tomato
puree, cinnamon, ginger, garlic, soy sauce, salt and pepper.
Then pour in the boiled water and mix it all together.
Bring to the boil over a medium heat, then reduce to a simmer.
Place a lid on the saucepan and let simmer for around 30 minutes.
Stir the courgettes (zucchini) into the pan along with the cannellini
beans and lime juice.
Simmer for another 30 minutes until the carrots are soft.
Serve with brown rice.

Low-fat roast dinner (yes, really)

This is basically what it says on the tin – a roast dinner without using much fat. Let's be real here – it won't be *quite* the same as your usual roast dinner, but it's close enough to make you feel like you're not missing out too much.

Ingredients

- chicken breast, skinless
- potatoes
- selection of vegetables – broccoli, cauliflower, green beans etc
- roasted vegetables (see recipe on page 101)
- herby roasted potatoes (see recipe on page 102)
- fat-free gravy (see recipe on page 103)
- optional: cauliflower cheese (see recipe on page 104)

Method

Pre-heat oven to 200°C/400°F.

Season the chicken breast with salt and pepper, wrap in foil and bake in the oven for 40 minutes or until cooked.

Meanwhile, prepare your roast potatoes, roasted veg and cauliflower cheese.

Boil or steam your chosen veg.

Make the gravy.

Serve them all together.

Other dinner ideas

Baked salmon with sweet potato mash and vegetables.

Grilled chicken breast with baked potato and tomato salad (see page 108 for dressings).

Grilled turkey breast with brown rice and green beans.

Vegan sausages with sweet potato mash and baked beans. ⭐

Grilled or baked cod with sweet potato 'fries' (see page 105).

Baked potato with baked beans and salad (see page 108 for dressings). ⭐⭐

Wholegrain pasta with tomato sauce. ⭐⭐

SIDE DISHES

Almost fat-free roasted vegetables

Ingredients

- new potatoes
- parsnips, peeled and quartered
- carrots, peeled and sliced into chunks
- sweet potatoes, peeled and cubed
- 2 purple or golden beets, peeled and halved
- salt and pepper
- rosemary (optional – for garnish)
- coconut or olive oil cooking spray, or wine / water for steam frying

Method

Pre-heat the oven to 200°C/400°F.

Place a roasting tin in the oven to heat up.

Place all your veg in a bowl and mix together with salt, pepper and the rosemary (if desired).

Remove the roasting tray from the oven and thinly coat the base with the cooking oil spray (or wine/water).

Add the veg to the tray and give it a few stirs to mix everything up.

Roast for 35-45 minutes, stirring halfway through.

Herby roast potatoes ✪✪✪

Ingredients

- coconut or olive oil spray,
- 4 cloves garlic
- mixed herbs
- potatoes, halved
- pinch of salt & pepper
- parsley and/or rosemary (optional for garnish)

Method

Peel and halve the potatoes, put them in a pan of boiling water and gently boil for around 15 minutes.

Meanwhile, heat a roasting pan in the oven (around 200°C/400°F).

Drain the potatoes, return them to the pan, put on a lid and give them a good, vigorous shake to roughen up the edges.

Take the pan from the oven, give it a thin coating of the oil spray, then add the potatoes along with the garlic and herbs.

Throw in some salt and pepper, give it all a good toss and then return to the oven.

After around 25 minutes, turn the potatoes, return them to the oven and roast them until they look good enough to eat.

Sprinkle with the parsley and/or rosemary if using.

Fat-free gravy ✪✪✪

Ingredients

- 4 tbsp gluten-free flour
- 1 tsp onion powder
- ½ tsp garlic powder
- 1 tsp mustard, English or Dijon
- pinch of salt and pepper
- 1 organic vegetable stock cube dissolved in 2 cups boiling water (broth)
- 2 tbsp Marmite, red wine or soy sauce (optional, to add flavour according to your tastes)

Method

Whisk the dry ingredients together over a medium-low heat until they become toasty – no more than a few minutes.

Slowly add the veg broth and whisk to remove any lumps.

Now add the mustard and/or optional ingredients and continue to stir.

Continue stirring over a medium-low heat until the gravy is bubbly and thickened.

Cheating cauliflower cheese ✪✪

Ingredients

- 1 cauliflower, washed and chopped into florets
- 250 ml (1 cup) boiling water
- 4 tbsp packet cheese-sauce granules – made with low-fat milk

Method

Cook the cauliflower in boiling water, or steam, for around 10 minutes, then drain and put it into an ovenproof dish.

Make up the cheese sauce according to the instructions, using skimmed milk.

Pour the sauce over the cooked cauliflower and mix well.

Add salt and pepper.

Place under a hot grill for 5-10 minutes until brown and bubbly.

Crispy oven-baked sweet potato fries ✪✪✪

Ingredients

- 7-8 sweet potatoes (medium)
- 1 tbs flour
- 1 tsp garlic powder
- 1 tsp onion powder
- 1 tsp paprika
- 1 tsp chilli powder
- salt and pepper to taste

Method

Clean and slice the potatoes into fairly thick chips/French fries.
Add to a pot of cold water (enough to cover them) and bring to the boil.
Boil for 5 minutes.
Pre-heat the oven to 200°C/400°F.
Line a roasting tray with parchment paper.
After boiling, drain the potatoes and place them back in the pot.
Add all the seasonings, cover and shake to distribute them.
Spread the chips evenly on the parchment-lined baking tray and bake for 20-25 minutes.

Roasted maple sprouts ✪✪✪

Ingredients

- 200 grams (2 cups) Brussels sprouts
- 8 new potatoes
- 1 tsp chilli flakes
- coconut or olive oil cooking spray or water/wine for steam frying
- salt and pepper
- 4 tbsp pomegranate seeds
- 2 tbsp maple syrup

Method

Pre-heat the oven to 200°C/400°F.

Halve the sprouts lengthways.

Cut the potatoes into pieces similar in size to the sprouts.

Place the sprouts and potatoes into a baking dish with the chilli flakes, spray 5-6 pumps of the cooking oil spray or water/wine over them, add salt and pepper and mix together.

Bake for 35-40 minutes until they start to turn a golden brown.

Take out of the oven, add the pomegranate seeds and toss.

Drizzle the maple syrup over the mixture and mix everything together.

Low-fat dumplings ✪

Ingredients

- 100 grams ($^7/_8$ cup) plain flour
- 1 tbsp baking powder
- 1 tsp caster sugar
- ½ tsp salt
- 1 tbsp butter
- 100 ml (½ cup) skimmed milk
- parsley (optional)

Method

In a medium-sized bowl, stir together the flour, baking powder, sugar and salt. Rub the butter into the mixture using your fingers, until crumbly.

Stir milk into the crumbed mixture to make a soft dough.

Drop by spoonfuls into boiling water.

Cover and simmer for 15 minutes without lifting the lid.

Serve immediately while piping hot.

Top tip: To make parsley dumplings, add 1 tablespoon chopped parsley to the dry ingredients

Salad dressings ✪✪✪

Yes, it is possible to have a healthy salad dressing. No oils required!

I deliberately haven't listed amounts because it's a case of trial and error – mix it up, taste it, add whatever is needed.

Here are a few ideas to help you on your creative journey – and it's okay to add a little olive oil, according to your own preference/tolerance.

The limey

Lime juice, chilli flakes, garlic

Sweet and tangy

Lemon juice, garlic, honey, mustard

Seeds of change

Pomegranate seeds, lemon juice, honey

The sweet ginger

Grated ginger, honey, lime juice

Dreamy creamy

Fat-free yoghurt, lemon juice, salt and pepper

Chilli lime supreme

Red pepper flakes, lime juice, soy sauce

Simple honey mustard

Mustard, honey, apple cider vinegar, salt and pepper

Ballsy balsamic

Balsamic vinegar, Dijon mustard, garlic, honey, salt and pepper

Lemon vinaigrette

Red wine vinegar, Dijon mustard, lemon juice and lemon zest, minced garlic, salt and pepper, mixed herbs to taste

My darling Clementine

Juice and zest of clementines, honey, apple cider vinegar, Dijon mustard, crushed garlic, salt and pepper

Top tip:
You can mix up a combination of any of these ingredients

DESSERTS

Remember when indulging your sweet tooth, if you have one (as I do), that it is easy to compensate for fat with sugar. But sugar must be kept to a minimum in the gallstone-friendly diet (as in all eating plans). This includes fructose (fruit sugar) which is turned straight into fat in the liver, and which can contribute to gallstones. So beware, and be aware.

Also, remember to stay away from cream, butter and nuts because of their high fat levels.

Fruit kebabs ✪✪✪

Ingredients/equipment

* Selection of fruit of your choice: works well with pineapple, berries, melon, blueberries, grapes, kiwi, raspberries.
* Skewers

Method

Slice your fruit into bite-size chunks.
Thread onto skewers.
Dust with a little sugar if required.

Top tip: Serve with fat-free yoghurt for dipping – scrumptious!

Baked apple ✪✪✪

Ingredients

- 4 cooking apples, cored but left whole
- 2 ginger stems, finely chopped
- ½ tsp ground cinnamon
- 4 prunes, chopped
- 50 grams (¼ cup) light muscovado sugar
- 2 tbsp honey

Method

Heat the oven to 200°C/400°F.

Using a sharp knife, score a line around the equator of each apple.

Put the scored apples into a baking dish with a small splash of water in the bottom.

In a bowl, combine the ginger, cinnamon, prunes and sugar.

Stuff this mixture into the apples so that they are well packed.

Cook for 30 minutes until soft and then remove from the oven.

Drizzle a little honey onto the apples and then return them to the oven for 5-10 minutes.

To test, pierce with a sharp knife – it should slide straight through.

Remove from the oven and baste the apples with the liquid left in the dish.

Serve hot with low-fat custard (see recipe opposite).

Low-fat custard ⭐⭐

Ingredients

- 600 ml (2 cups) skimmed milk
- 2 egg whites
- 2 tbsp cornflour
- 100 grams (½ cup) caster sugar
- 1 tsp vanilla extract
- 1 banana (optional for serving)

Method

Heat the milk on the stove in a saucepan, until it is almost boiling.
Whilst the milk is warming, whisk up the 2 egg whites with the cornflour and sugar until lump free.
When the milk is almost boiling, add it to the bowl of egg mixture and stir.
Pour it all back into the saucepan and heat gently for a couple of minutes whilst stirring all the time, until it thickens (depending on how thick you like your custard).
Once it is the desired consistency, just add the vanilla extract and stir in.
Serve with sliced bananas.

Nearly no-fat banana bread ✪✪

Ingredients

- coconut or olive oil cooking spray
- 200 grams (1½ cups) gluten-free, whole-wheat flour
- 140 grams (¾ cup) caster sugar
- 1¼ tsp baking powder
- ½ tsp bicarbonate of soda/baking soda
- ½ tsp ground cinnamon
- 2 egg whites
- 3 ripe bananas, mashed
- 4 tbsp apple sauce

Method

Pre-heat the oven to 180°C/350°F.

Lightly grease a 20x10 cm (8x4 in) loaf tin with a few pumps of the cooking spray.

In a large bowl, stir together flour, sugar, baking powder, bicarbonate of soda (baking soda) and cinnamon.

Add the egg whites, bananas and apple purée and stir just until combined.

Pour the batter into the prepared tin.

Bake in the pre-heated oven for 50 to 55 minutes, until a skewer inserted into the centre of the loaf comes out clean.

Turn out onto a wire rack and allow to cool before slicing.

Top tip: If your bananas are already black but you can't make a cake right away, simply pop them in the freezer. Defrost the bananas whenever you're ready to bake

Chocolate brownies ✪

Ingredients

- coconut or olive oil cooking spray
- 128 grams (1 cup) gluten-free flour
- 35 grams (1/3 cup) unsweetened cocoa powder
- ½ tsp salt
- ½ tsp baking powder
- ¼ tsp bicarbonate of soda / baking soda
- ¼ tsp ground cinnamon
- 125 grams (½ cup) brown sugar
- 30g (¼ cup) fat-free dry milk powder
- 1 egg white, slightly beaten
- 255 grams (1 cup) unsweetened apple sauce (recipe on page 56)
- 1 tsp vanilla extract
- 1 tsp powdered sugar for dusting (optional)

Method

Pre-heat the oven to 180°C/350°F.

Lightly coat a 20x10 cm (8x4 in) baking pan with cooking spray and then set it aside.

In a large bowl, sift together the flour, unsweetened cocoa, salt, baking powder, bicarbonate of soda (baking soda) and cinnamon until well mixed, then set the bowl aside.

In a medium bowl, beat together the sugar, fat-free dry milk powder, egg white, applesauce and vanilla extract with a spoon until well combined.

Stir the wet mixture into the dry mixture, mixing just until the ingredients are well moistened. Do not over mix – once they are moist, stop mixing.

Spread the brownie batter evenly in the prepared baking pan and bake in the oven for 20 to 25 minutes or until a toothpick inserted in the centre comes out clean.

Cool on a wire rack and give the brownies a light dusting with powdered sugar, if desired.

Fruit sorbet ✪✪✪

Ingredients

- 1.4 kg (4 cups) prepared fruit (see below) cut into pieces
- 2-4 tbsp sugar
- 1/2 small lemon, juice of
- 1/2 small lime, juice of

Suggested combinations:
- mango and strawberries
- bananas and strawberries
- pineapple and bananas
- pineapple and mango

Method

Prepare the fruit by peeling, if necessary, and cutting it into chunks.
Place the chunks on a plate or tray covered with plastic wrap or equivalent, making sure everything is as spread out as possible.
Freeze overnight.
The next morning, take the fruit from the freezer and whizz it through a food processor until very finely chopped.
Add the sugar and lemon juice, adjusting either according to the sweetness and acidity levels of the fruit you are working with and your preferences; if you use pineapple, use orange juice or water instead of lemon or lime juice and add a little vanilla extract if necessary.
Taste the mixture in case it needs adjusting.
Blend thoroughly until very smooth, scraping down the sides of the food processor regularly; this may take up to five minutes.
Spoon into serving dishes or a covered storage tub and return to the freezer until it is time to serve the sorbet.
Put in the fridge to temper 15 minutes before serving.

Other dessert ideas

Banana custard (page 114)

Fat-free yoghurt with honey

Fat-free yoghurt with fruit

Fruit salad

Shop-bought sorbet, but this can be very sweet (so watch sugar content)

Alpro soya desserts

Shop-bought fruit bars

Low-fat popcorn

SNACKS

Top tip

It would seem that it is a good idea to give your gut a rest in between meals, but if you must snack, it is a good idea to stick to small, healthy snacks that won't put too much pressure on your gallbladder in between meals.

Suggestions for snacking

Raw veg

Served with fat-free yoghurt dip or salsa

Frozen grapes

Place washed grapes in the freezer for at least 2 hours

Honeyed yogurt

Bowl of fat-free Greek yoghurt with a dash of cinnamon and 1 tsp honey

Grilled pineapple

Put a few slices of fresh pineapple under the grill, or 'flash-fry' them in a couple of sprays of cooking spray

Citrus berry salad

Bowl of mixed berries (raspberries, strawberries, blueberries, and / or blackberries) tossed with 1 tbsp freshly squeezed orange juice

Vanilla and banana smoothie

One sliced banana, a tub of fat-free vanilla Greek yoghurt, and a handful of ice – blend until smooth

Banana chips

One small banana sliced, dipped in lemon juice and baked until crisp

Fruity soft serve

Purée a small frozen banana; this comes up like ice cream. You can add berries if desired.

Café latte

Steamed skimmed milk with a shot of espresso

Kale chips

A bunch of raw kale (stems removed) sprayed with cooking oil spray and baked at 200°C/400°F until crispy

Crunchy kale salad

A bunch of chopped kale leaves tossed with 1 tsp honey and 1 tbsp balsamic vinegar

Strawberry salad

A bunch of raw spinach mixed with a handful of sliced strawberries and a tbsp of balsamic vinegar

BEVERAGES

The ginger mix ✪✪✪

Ginger is cleansing, refreshing, detoxifying and really good for your gut, but it can also aggravate gallstones, so watch your intake of ginger and consult a doctor if you are concerned. I have included this recipe because it is a good option for a post-surgery drink. Introduce it into your diet gradually though.

Ingredients

- 2 litres filtered water
- 10 slices fresh, peeled ginger
- 2 sliced organic lemons
- half a cucumber
- mint

Method

Mix all ingredients together.
Strain before drinking.

Ginger tea ✪✪✪

Ingredients

- 10-15 slices fresh, peeled ginger (but see note about ginger in previous recipe)
- 1.5 litres filtered water
- juice of 2 organic lemons

Method

Boil the water in a pan and add the ginger.
Simmer for 20 minutes.
Add the lemon juice.
Sip throughout the day.

Lemon water ✪✪✪

Ingredients

- juice of 4 organic lemons
- 1.5 litres filtered water

Method

Squeeze the lemon juice into the water and sip throughout the day. (Be mindful lemon is acidic and can be hard on tooth enamel so vary this with other drinks.)

Raw vegetable juice ✪✪✪

Ingredients

- 1 large beetroot
- 8 beetroot leaves
- 8 endive leaves
- 2 stalks celery
- ¼ red onion
- 1 large carrot
- 2 red radishes
- 1 small apple

Method

Juice all the ingredients and drink immediately.
(This makes a good breakfast juice and is an excellent way to start the day.)

Water!

If you don't feel like bothering with the above, make sure you are drinking at least 2 litres of water a day.

A note about alcohol and gallstones

As I have already said, I drank all the way through my gallstones, and it didn't harm them, or me, in any way. You may take a different approach, and you probably should too, but for other reasons around alcohol being a risk factor for many ailments.

Interestingly enough, and definitely worth mentioning here: I discovered during my research that some observational studies* claim that people who totally abstain from drinking alcohol can be more prone to developing gallstones.

The bottom line – don't take my advice in this regard.

---

* Wang J, Duan X, Li B, Jiang X. Alcohol consumption and risk of gallstone disease: a meta-analysis. *European Journal of Gastroenterology & Hepatology* 2017;29(4) :e19-e28. doi: 10.1097/MEG.0000000000000803. PubMed PMID: 27926662.

SANS-GALLBLADDER
Recipes and tips

When the 'problem' has been removed, it is tempting to go back to eating a similar diet to the one that got you into trouble in the first place. But really, it's best not to. For a start (you know what I'm going to say), go easy on the fat because you can no longer deliver large amounts of bile to digest it. In particular:

- avoid fried, greasy food or anything containing hydrogenated fat (e.g. margarine, crisps)
- limit refined sugar intake
- avoid a high-carb diet
- eat plenty of fibre, especially from vegetables
- eat smaller meals, more frequently
- eat plenty of food containing essential fatty acids - for instance, fish and other seafood (especially cold-water fatty fish, such as salmon, mackerel, tuna, herring and sardines); nuts and seeds.

The goal is to re-introduce healthy fats back into your diet, but you should still be aware of fat, sugar and carb content.

My favourite recipes

Now that I am not terrified of fat, I have adapted my diet to include meals containing healthy fats; see a few examples in the following pages.

Beetroot salad

Ingredients

- 6 medium beetroot, cut into quarters
- 3 tbsp (¼ cup) extra-virgin olive oil
- 2 tbsp white-wine vinegar
- ½ tsp Dijon mustard
- ½ tsp honey
- ½ tsp salt
- freshly ground pepper, to taste
- 1 large shallot, finely chopped
- 1 stalk celery, finely chopped

Method

Pre-heat the oven to 200°C/400°F.

Divide the beetroot between two pieces of foil; bring the edges together and crimp to make packets. Roast until the beetroots are is just tender when pierced with the point of a knife – about 1¼ hours.

Unwrap the beetroot and allow to cool.

Meanwhile, whisk the olive oil, vinegar, mustard, honey, salt and pepper in a small bowl to make a dressing.

When the beetroots are cool enough to handle, slip off the skins.

Cut them into small cubes and place in a large bowl.

Add the shallots, celery and dressing; toss to coat well.

Serve at room temperature or chilled.

Veggie Buddha bowl

Ingredients

- 225 grams (1¼ cups) short-grain brown rice or long-grain brown rice, rinsed
- 200 grams (1½ cups) frozen shelled edamame, preferably organic
- 200 grams (1½ cups) trimmed and roughly chopped snap peas or snow peas, or thinly sliced broccoli florets
- 1 to 2 tbsp reduced-sodium tamari or soy sauce, to taste
- 280 grams (4 cups) of any of the following: chopped red cabbage, spinach, romaine lettuce or kale (ribs removed)
- 2 ripe avocados, halved, pitted and thinly sliced into long strips (slice just before serving)

Garnish with all or some of:
- 1 small cucumber, thinly sliced
- thinly sliced spring onion (green onion) – about ½ small bunch)
- lime wedges
- toasted sesame oil, for drizzling
- sesame seeds
- sea salt and pepper
- any dressing of your choice

Method

Bring a large pot of water to the boil.

Once the water is boiling, add the rice and continue boiling for 25 minutes.

Add the edamame and cook for 3 more minutes (it's okay if the water doesn't reach a rapid boil again), then add the snap peas and cook for 2 more minutes.

Drain well, and return the rice and veg to the pot.

Season to taste with 1 to 2 tablespoons of tamari or soy sauce, and stir to combine.

Divide the rice/veg mixture and raw veg into 4 bowls.

Arrange cucumber slices along the edges of the bowls.

Drizzle lightly with a dressing of your choice and top with sliced spring (green) onion.

Place a lime wedge or two in each bowl.

When you're ready to serve, divide the avocado into the bowls.

Lightly drizzle sesame oil over the avocado, followed by a generous sprinkling of sesame seeds and sea salt.

Serve immediately.

Salmon, avocado and lemon salad

Ingredients

- 1 piece of salmon fillet
- ½ avocado, cubed
- ¼ cucumber, cubed
- ½ head of lettuce
- 1 lemon
- 1 tbsp chopped chives
- salt and pepper

Method

Season the salmon and grill for 5 minutes, until cooked.

Put the avocado and cucumber into a bowl and add the lettuce.

Peel the lemon and squeeze half of its juice onto the salad, then add a couple of lemon slices.

Peel the skin from the salmon and flake it onto the salad.

Sprinkle on the chives and squeeze on more lemon to taste.

Add salt and pepper to taste.

Salmon bake

Ingredients

- 1 salmon fillet
- 2 tbsp melted butter
- ½ lemon
- salt and pepper
- olive oil cooking spray

For the crumb topping:
- ¾ cup Panko bread crumbs
- 3 cloves garlic, minced
- 2 tbsp fresh parsley, chopped
- 1 tbsp fresh dill, chopped
- zest from one lemon
- 2 tbsp parmesan cheese, shredded
- 3 tbsp melted butter

Method

Pre-heat the oven to 200°C/400°F.
Combine all the ingredients for the crumb topping in a small bowl.
Line a pan with foil and lightly spray with cooking oil spray.
Place the salmon in the pan and brush with the melted butter.
Season with salt and pepper and squeeze the lemon over the top.
Sprinkle the crumb topping mixture over the salmon.
Bake uncovered for around 15 minutes or until the salmon flakes
    easily and is cooked through.

Chilli chicken wrap

Ingredients

- 2 tbsp olive oil
- 6 boneless, skinless chicken thighs, cut into bite-sized pieces
- 1 large onion, thinly sliced into half-moons
- 2 garlic cloves, finely chopped
- 3 cm (1 inch) piece ginger, peeled and finely chopped
- sea salt (pinch)
- ½ tsp ground cumin
- ½ tsp garam masala
- 1 tbsp tomato purée
- 1 red chilli, thinly sliced into rings
- juice ½ lemon
- 4 rotis, warmed
- ½ small red onion, chopped
- 4 tbsp mango chutney or lime pickle
- 4 tbsp yoghurt

Method

Heat the olive oil in a large frying pan over a medium heat.
Add the chicken, brown on all sides, then remove.
Add the onion, garlic, ginger and a pinch of salt, then cook for 5 minutes or until softened.
Increase the heat to high.
Return the chicken to the pan with the spices, tomato purée, chilli and lemon juice, then season well and cook for 10 minutes or until the chicken is tender.
Divide the chicken, red onion, chutney, herbs and yoghurt between the four warm rotis.
Roll up and serve.

Fish tacos

Ingredients

- 220 grams (½ lb) lemon sole fillets
- olive oil cooking spray
- salt and freshly ground black pepper
- 1 tsp chipotle paste
- 6 tbsp mayonnaise
- 4 soft corn tortillas
- 175 grams (1¾ cups) white cabbage, shredded
- handful coriander (cilantro), chopped
- 1 small red onion, finely chopped
- juice of 1 small lime, plus lime wedges to serve (optional)

Method

Heat the oven to 200°C/400°F.

Space the sole fillets apart on a baking sheet, spray with a little olive oil spray, sprinkle with salt and pepper, and bake for 12-15 minutes

Meanwhile, mix the chipotle paste into the mayo and warm the tortillas.

To make the salad, toss the cabbage, coriander (cilantro) and onion with the lime juice and some salt.

Spread the tortillas with a little of the spicy mayo, then place the salad and fish down the centre.

Top with a little more mayo, then fold and eat with your fingers.

Serve with lime wedges.

Sweet potato and black bean burger

Ingredients

For the burgers:

- 170 grams (1 cup) quinoa
- 2 medium-sweet potatoes, halved lengthwise
- olive oil spray
- ¼ tsp salt
- 1 tsp onion powder
- ½ tsp garlic powder
- 1 tsp chilli powder
- ¼ tsp dried oregano
- 2 tsp cumin powder
- ¼ tsp black pepper
- 1 x 400 gram (14 oz) can black beans, drained and rinsed
- wholegrain burger buns or lettuce wraps
- lettuce, tomatoes, avocados

For the chilli lime mayo:

- 230 grams (¼ cup) mayonnaise
- 1 tsp chilli garlic sauce
- juice of ¼ lime

Method

Pre-heat the oven to 200°C/400°F.

Cook the quinoa according to the instructions on the package. Cover and set aside.

Place the sweet potato halves on a baking tray, cut side down, coat lightly with olive oil spray and roast for 30 minutes.

While the sweet potatoes are baking, make the chilli lime mayo: in a small bowl, mix together the mayo, chilli garlic sauce and lime juice; set aside.

In another small bowl, mix together salt, onion powder, garlic powder, chilli powder, oregano, cumin powder and black pepper, then set aside.

In a large bowl, add the black beans and cooked sweet potatoes and mash until the consistency is slightly chunky – some beans will be completely mashed and others will not, creating a nice texture.

Add in the cooked quinoa and spices, mix together with your hands and form into 8 burger patties – about 1/3 cup of mixture each.

Place the burger patties on a large baking sheet covered in parchment paper, then spray with olive oil and bake for 20 minutes.

Flip over, spray the other side with olive oil spray and bake for a further 10 minutes.

Serve with a wholegrain burger bun and salad, or wrapped in a lettuce leaf.

Spicy chicken, spinach and sweet potato casserole

Ingredients

- 3 sweet potatoes, cut into chunks
- 225 grams (1 cup) spinach
- 1 tbsp olive oil
- 8 chicken thighs, skinless and boneless
- 500 ml (2¼ cups) chicken stock

For the spice paste:
- 2 onions, chopped
- 1 red chilli, chopped
- 1 tsp paprika
- 1 small piece of fresh ginger, grated
- 1 x 400 gram (14 oz) can tomatoes
- 2 lemons, deseeded and chopped

To serve:
- pumpkin seeds, toasted
- 2-3 lemons, de-seeded and chopped
- 4 warm naan

Method

Steam the sweet potatoes: Place a steamer basket in a wide, shallow pan with a lid; place washed sweet potatoes into the steamer basket; fill the pan with water up to the bottom of the steamer basket; season the sweet potatoes: cover the pan and bring the water to a boil; reduce the heat slightly and let the potatoes steam for 20 to 30 minutes, depending on their size. This works best with smaller potatoes.

Meanwhile, put all the paste ingredients in a food processor and blend until very finely chopped; set aside.

Put the spinach in a large colander in the sink and pour the water from the steamer pan over it to wilt the spinach; leave to steam-dry.

Return the pan to the heat, add the oil followed by the spice paste, then fry the paste for about 5 minutes until thickened.

Add the chicken and fry for 8-10 minutes until the chicken starts to colour.

Pour over the stock, bring to the boil and leave to simmer for 10 minutes, stirring occasionally.

Check the chicken is cooked by cutting into one of the thighs and making sure it's white throughout with no signs of pink.

Season with black pepper, then add the sweet potato.

Leave to simmer for a further 5 minutes.

Meanwhile, roughly chop the spinach and add it to the stew.

Scatter over the pumpkin seeds and lemons, and serve with warm naan.

Lettuce wraps with black beans and quinoa

Ingredients

- 170 grams (1 cup) uncooked quinoa
- 1 Romaine lettuce, whole leaves torn off
- 1 x 400 gram (14 oz) can black beans, drained and rinsed
- 1 x 400 gram (14 oz) can sweetcorn, drained and rinsed
- juice of 1 lime
- 1 tsp cumin
- 1 tsp paprika powder
- 15 grams (½ cup) fresh parsley, chopped
- 2 spring (green) onions, sliced
- 250 grams (1 cup) white bean spread or hummus
- sea salt
- black pepper
- red pepper flakes
- hot sauce (optional)

Method

Cook the quinoa according to the instructions on the package.
In a bowl, combine the black beans and the corn with the quinoa, lime juice, cumin, paprika powder and chopped parsley.
Season with salt, pepper, and red pepper flakes.
Equally apportion the quinoa mixture to the lettuce leaves and top them with some hummus, spring (green) onions, and hot sauce if you fancy.
Add cooked chicken if you so desire.

Aubergine and lentil bake

Ingredients

- 2 aubergines, cut into slices lengthways
- 3 tbsp olive oil
- 140 grams (5/8 cup) Puy lentils
- 2 onions, finely chopped
- 3 garlic cloves, chopped
- 300 grams (1½ cups) cooked butternut squash
- 1 x 400 gram (14 oz) can chopped tomatoes
- handful basil leaves
- salt and pepper
- 125 gram (1 cup) mozzarella, torn

Method

Heat the oven to 200°C/400°F.
Brush both sides of the aubergine slices with 2 tbsp of the olive oil, lay on a baking sheet, season and bake for 15-20 minutes until tender, turning once.
Cook the lentils following the instructions on the packet.
Heat the remaining oil in a large frying pan.
Add the onions and garlic and cook until soft.
Stir through the squash and tomatoes, plus ½ can of water.
Simmer for 10-15 minutes until the sauce has thickened.
Stir in the lentils, basil and seasoning.
Spoon a layer of lentils into a small baking dish.
Top with some of the aubergine slices and repeat, finishing with a layer of aubergine.
Scatter with the pieces of mozzarella and bake for a further 15 minutes until the cheese is golden and bubbling.

APPENDICES

Gallbladder disease and nutrition
Interview with an expert

During the course of researching and writing this book, I came across some differing views and opinions with regard to nutrition. In an effort to gain some clarity, I spoke to naturopath Margaret Jasinska, ND, who co-wrote *Save Your Gallbladder and what to do if you've already lost it.*

Below is a snippet of our conversation:

Alcohol

Question: I read that a person who abstains from alcohol is shown to be at greater risk of developing gallstones. Is that something to be concerned about?

Answer: This would have been an observational study, which doesn't prove causation.

Question: I also read (and we all know) that alcohol is not conducive to optimal health. What is your opinion on this?

Answer: Alcohol can raise triglycerides and increase the risk of a fatty liver, both of which pre-dispose us to gallbladder problems.

Grains

Question: In your book, you recommend staying away from grains, but also that fibre intake is important. So in your opinion, would the total abstinence from wholegrain pasta, bread and rice be advised as part of a 'gallstone-friendly' or 'post-gallbladder-removal' diet?

Answer: Yes. There is abundant fibre in vegetables, nuts and seeds so it is important to eat these daily. The fibre in those foods is less likely to irritate the gut lining than the fibre, lectins and saponins in grains.

Coffee

Question: A few studies have shown that consuming coffee in moderation can be beneficial to a gallstone sufferer. Do you agree?

Answer: Yes. Moderate coffee consumption is beneficial for liver health and coffee does promote bile secretion.

Eggs

Question: I have read multiple times that eggs can be harmful to a gallstone sufferer, yet I have also read that eggs provide essential protein as well as vitamins and nutrients. What is your take on eggs?

Answer: Egg intolerance is common among people with a gallbladder condition and many of our gallbladder patients are more symptomatic when they eat eggs.

Supplements

Question: If you could recommend ONE single supplement for a gallstone sufferer to take, what would it be and why?

Answer: St Mary's thistle (also known as milk thistle – see page 44) because it improves the health of the liver – helping it to produce better quality bile, which is higher in bile salts (that is, thinner bile that is less likely to form stones).

Question: Would this be different for someone who has had their gallbladder removed?

Answer: Those individuals would also greatly benefit from St Mary's thistle because they are at risk of stones forming in the bile ducts within their liver, and also of fatty liver.

Fructose

Question: In your book you say that fruit should be limited to twice a day by anyone wishing to lose weight or dissolve gallstones, due to fructose levels. Would this apply to someone who has already lost their gallbladder?

Answer: Yes, due to risk of developing gallstones in the bile ducts inside the liver, and fatty liver.

Question: Would you advocate limiting fruit intake generally by, say, a person who does not need to lose weight or does not wish to dissolve gallstones (if, say, they were waiting for the operation)?

Answer: Yes. The diet should contain abundant vegetables, as they are high in vitamins, minerals and fibre, and low in sugar, unlike fruit.

Meat

Question: I found very little mention of meat (white or red) in my research. In your opinion, is a vegetarian more or less likely to develop gallstones? Would you recommend cutting down or cutting out meat from a healthy diet, regardless of the 'ethics' of vegetarianism?

Answer: My opinion is that meat is a healthy food to include in the diet and that flour, sugar and alcohol are unhealthy foods. It depends on the context of the overall diet – meat with broccoli is a healthy meal (not meat with pasta, wine and then dessert).

Cholesterol

Question: When I had gallstones, I altered my diet to cut down on fat – for instance, I ate a lot of prawns once I realised they are low in fat. But now I realise I should have been looking more at the cholesterol content. Do you agree?

Answer: The cholesterol content of food has negligible effects on blood cholesterol levels. Sugar, grains, cereals, starches and alcohol raise insulin levels, and insulin then instructs the liver to manufacture cholesterol. So eliminating those foods is key.

And lastly...

Question: What would you say to someone who has been diagnosed with gallstones and told they need surgery, who wishes to explore alternative options, but is scared of the intense pain associated with gallstone attacks? For instance, after diagnosis and prior to the op, I did read about dissolving stones/flushing them out, but as soon as I saw that olive oil was involved, I was too scared to try it, knowing that olive oil was one of my triggers.

Answer: Sometimes surgery is the only option – for example, if the patient is in frequent pain, the gallbladder is inflamed or infected, the pancreas is inflamed, etc. If none of those factors applies, it is best to work on slowly dissolving gallstones, which usually takes a few years.

Recommended reading

I think I may have already said this, and yet, here I go again: I am not an expert. I am more of an unwilling participant in the gallstone epidemic – one who happens to have felt the need to compile a book of recipes which might help fellow sufferers. If you are looking for more detailed information about the gallbladder, gallstones, diet or treatment, please see the following recommended reading:

Dr Sandra Cabot MD and Margaret Jasinska ND. *Save Your Gallbladder and what to do if you've already lost it.* 2013. SCB (Sarah Cabot Books) International.

Dr Sarah Brewer. *Overcoming Gallstones: nutritional, medical and surgical approaches.* 2014. Createspace/Medilance.

Monika Shah. *The Gallbladder Diet Guide: A Complete Diet Guide for People with Gallbladder Disorders* (Gallbladder Diet, Gallbladder Removal Diet, Flush Techniques, Yoga's, Mudras & Home Remedies for Instant Pain Relief). 2017: Createspace.

Further research notes

I realise that there are those of you who would like some real *facts*, not just my largely uneducated opinion, though I have included excerpts from books written by people far more educated than I. (With their permission, of course).

However, in my research for this book, I did come across facts, research papers and references, which do not necessarily fit with the tone of this book but may provide some further (intelligent) information. Enjoy!

Cholelithiasis: Noun meaning the formation of gallstones.

Cholecystectomy: Noun meaning the surgical removal of the gallbladder.

Asymptomatic cholelithiasis: is cholecystectomy really needed?

To quote from the paper by Sakorafas et al: 'About 10-20% of people in most western countries have gallstones, and among them 50-70% are asymptomatic at the time of diagnosis. Despite some controversy, most authors agree that the vast majority of these people should be managed by observation alone ("expectant management"). Routine cholecystectomy for all subjects with silent gallstones is too aggressive a management option. Management options should be extensively discussed with the patient; he or she should be actively involved in the process of therapeutic decision making.'

Sakorafas GH, Milingos D, Peros G. Asymptomatic cholelithiasis: is cholecystectomy really needed? A critical reappraisal 15 years after the introduction of laparoscopic cholecystectomy. *Dig Dis Sci* 2007; 52(5): 1313–1325.

Gallstone formation during weight-reduction dieting

To quote from the abstract of Liddle et al: 'A study was undertaken involving 51 obese subjects, who were put on calorie-controlled diets, and 26 non-dieting subjects. Over an 8 week period, the subjects (who were deemed to have no gallstones prior to the study) were scanned to investigate any formation of gallstones. Sonography performed after 4 weeks of dieting revealed new-onset gallbladder sludge in 1 subject and gallstones in 4 subjects. After 8 weeks of dieting, sludge was detected in 3 subjects and gallstones in 13 (25.5%). In contrast, none of the non-dieting subjects developed any detectable gallbladder abnormalities. During the dieting period, one of 51 subjects developed symptoms of biliary colic, necessitating cholecystectomy. On cessation of dieting with reinstitution of normal feeding, two additional subjects with stones developed symptoms severe enough to require cholecystectomy. It was concluded that this form of weight-reduction dieting predisposes to the development of gallstones and that gallstone formation is a risk of this type of prolonged calorie restriction.'

Liddle RA, Goldstein RB, Saxton J. Gallstone formation during weight-reduction dieting. *Arch Intern Med* 1989; 149: 1750–1753.

Gallstones and genetics

A study by Nakeeb et al concluded that genetic factors are responsible for at least 30% of symptomatic gallstone disease. However, the true role of heredity in gallstone pathogenesis is probably higher because data based on symptomatic gallbladder disease underestimates the true prevalence in the population.

Nakeeb A, Comuzzie AG, Martin L, Sonnenberg GE, Swartz-Basile D, Kissebah AH, Pitt HA. Gallstones: genetics versus environment. *Annals of Surgery* 2002; 235(6): 842–849.

To quote from the study by Wittenbury & Lammert: 'Geographic and ethnic differences in gallstone prevalence rates and familial clustering of cholelithiasis imply that genetic factors influence the risk of gallstone formation.'

Wittenburg H, Lammert F. Genetic predisposition to gallbladder stones. *Semin Liver Dis* 2007; 27(1): 109-121.

Can soluble dietary fibre protect against cholesterol gallstone formation?

Studies have shown that dietary soluble fibre inhibits cholesterol stone formation by reducing the biliary cholesterol saturation index. This protective effect is associated with a selective decrease in biliary cholesterol.

(Soluble fibre is found in oats, peas, beans, apples, citrus fruits, carrots, barley and psyllium.)

Schwesinger WH, Kurtin WE, Page CP, Stewart RM, Johnson R. Soluble dietary fiber protects against cholesterol gallstone formation. *American Journal of Surgery* 1999; 177: 307–310.

Can children get gallstones?

Yes, children can get gallstones and the occurrence of paediatric gallstones is increasing. In fact, a study conducted in 2012 concluded that there had been a three-fold increase in the incidence of paediatric cholecystectomy in England since 1997, with a particular rise among white females. Although data on BMI (body mass index) was not available, the observed effect may be a consequence of increasing levels of teenage obesity.

Khoo AK, Cartwright R, Berry S, Davenport M. Cholecystectomy in English children: evidence of an epidemic (1997-2012). *J Pediatr Surg* 2014; 49(2): 284-288. doi: 10.1016/j.jpedsurg.2013.11.053.

Index

Also available...

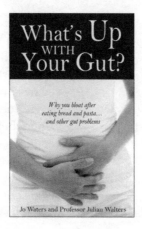

What's Up With Your Gut?

Why you bloat after eating bread and pasta... and other gut problems

By Jo Waters and Professor Julian Walters

What's Up With Your Gut? takes a practical look at the full range of gut problems, using a symptom-led approach so that sufferers can recognise what may have been troubling them for years and find solutions.

It then describes the range of solutions, both standard and alternative, emphasising the importance of what is eaten/food intolerances and the impact of poor digestion on overall health. Whether you suffer cramping diarrhoea when you are stressed out, get constipated when you're on holiday or just feel fatigued by your grumbling guts, they show what the options are for diagnosis, symptom improvement and tackling the underlying causes.

www.hammersmithbooks.co.uk/product/your-gut/